Praise for *Up Bow, Down Bow*

"Children with varying abilities have much to offer all of us. This book speaks to how parents, families, and communities can support children with diverse capabilities and the joy we can receive in return"
—Barbara Bowman, Irving B. Harris Professor, Erikson Institute

"This book is a must read for everyone. In eloquent prose Nancy and April share how music can give a voice to everyone and break down seemingly insurmountable barriers. The cello lessons in this book sing to the reader on so many levels. This book teaches that G-d sends all of us challenges and tests, and our job is to find the beauty and blessing hidden in those challenges. This is what Nancy and her husband have been able to do with their wonderful son, Alex, who was born with many disabilities. They chose to focus on the positive and what Alex can do, and that is the message to us all. What a blessing this is to anyone who reads it."
—Susie Garber, educator, mother, grandmother, reporter, speaker, and author.

"This remarkable book continues the story, begun in the wonderful *Up Not Down Syndrome,* of Alex, a boy with Trisomy 21 and an insatiable desire to learn and grow, and his mother, Nancy, a woman with an insatiable desire to see that Alex gets those learning and growing opportunities. Now Nancy teams with a remarkable young music educator, April Beard, to tell the story of Alex's introduction to the world of music through instruction in playing the cello. The story is beautifully and compellingly told through three voices, Nancy's, April's, and Alex's, as this trio navigates the challenges of achieving what some might see as an impossible task. In the end, this is a tale of the triumph of the human spirit. The triumph managed through a parent's love and persistence, a teacher's dedication, a young boy's desire to learn, and music's power to transform."
—Russ Walsh, Rider University, author of
A Parent's Guide to Public Education in the 21st Century

"You write so simply, so lucidly, yet so profoundly. This is, just exquisite."
—Brenda Dixon-Gottschild, Ph.D., author, lecturer, consultant, teacher, performer, and Prof. Emerita, Dance Studies, Temple University.

"It is thrilling to see Alex grow physically, emotionally, and mentally through learning the cello! The teamwork approach among Alex, April and Nancy is amazing. It's a miracle that music connects not only to our inner selves, but also to the people we share it with."
—Jennifer Jie Jin, cellist

"Schwartz and Beard's ability to work in tandem with one another, Schwartz as Alex's mother, Beard as Alex's teacher; show the power impact, perception and belief towards what children with varying abilities can do or will be able to do has on both their personal growth and quality of life. This collaboration offers a promising and powerful blueprint for educators, parents, and caregivers everywhere to collaborate, teach, and love all children within the space of strength-based perspectives."
—Kass Minor Co-Founding Educator and Executive Director, The Minor Collective

"*Up Bow, Down Bow: A Child with Down Syndrome and His Journey to Master the Cello* by Nancy M. Schwartz and April E. Beard is a multivocal learning narrative that weaves the rhythms of a mother's vision and persistence, a teacher's skill and dedication, a young boy's vitality and commitment to learning with the power of relational music instruction. In this book, the cello is a portal—to an illuminating vision of how families, educators, and communities can optimally support children with diverse capabilities in ways that generate reciprocal learning and transformation."
—Sharon M. Ravitch, Ph.D., University of Pennsylvania Graduate School of Education

"This book, co-authored by the kind of teacher or parent that every child deserves, captures the magical powers of music to meet learners where they are. It is a loving thank you note to every teacher whose lessons have built our competence and confidence. While it is the continuing and triumphant story of one child's journey towards independence, *Up Bow, Down Bow* is also a universal guide to how to live a good life—working together as a team and looking beyond obstacles to embrace new challenges."

—Betty Litsinger, Director of Multilingual Writing, Bryn Mawr College

"This beautiful book shows the inner beauty of a whole community, focused around the inner beauty of Alex, a little boy with Down syndrome. It is the joint account of a loving mother and a talented, loving music teacher in helping Alex to grow through learning to play the cello. At twelve years of age, Alex is unable to do many of the things we take for granted, including speech, and yet... Read, and be inspired."

—Bob Rich, PhD, professional grandfather and author of *From Depression to Contentment*

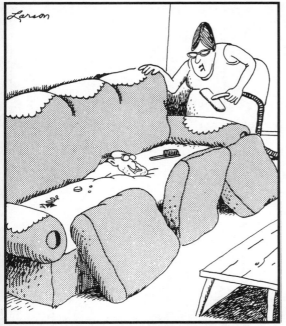

"Andrew! So that's where you've been! And good heavens! ... There's my old hairbrush, too!"

Larson

UP BOW DOWN BOW

A CHILD WITH DOWN SYNDROME AND HIS JOURNEY TO MASTER THE CELLO

NANCY M. SCHWARTZ
and APRIL E. BEARD

Modern History Press

Ann Arbor, MI

ISBN 978-1-61599-703-9 paperback
ISBN 978-1-61599-704-6 hardcover
ISBN 978-1-61599-705-3 eBook

Published by
Modern History Press   www.ModernHistoryPress.com
5145 Pontiac Trail   info@ModernHistoryPress.com
Ann Arbor, MI 48105   Tollfree 888-761-6268

Dedication

Nancy:

In memory of my dad, Martin Levine, my father-in-law, Lenny Schwartz, my mother-in-law, Sandy Schwartz, my mother, JoAnne Liebenberg Levine, and for Charlotte Figi who changed our world.

April:

For my parents: Thank you for your endless love, support, and energy.
And for every child who thinks they can't: You can!

"As you've discovered, so many things are possible
just as long as you don't know they are impossible."
Norton Juster, *The Phantom Tollbooth*

"For there is always light,
if only we are brave enough to see it.
If only we are brave enough to be it."
Amanda Gorman, *The Hill We Climb*

Contents

1   Nancy

My third son, Alex, has Down Syndrome. When he first arrived into our family—after the easiest of my three labors—I had no idea how blooming and bright he would be. I was scared. Everything about mothering Alex seemed like it would be uncharted territory, and I felt inadequate as well as sad.

What about all my dreams for who he'd be?

In the twelve years since Alex and I met, face-to-face for the first time, I have come to view him as a sunflower. Not just me, either. Our family and Alex's many friends see him always growing in the direction of light and love, the way a sunflower grows towards the sun.

It was in Alex's honor that my extraordinary first son, Alex's brother, Josh, drew "Sunflower." Josh's pictorial ode to his youngest brother shows a child's hand grasping a sunflower in the same way Alex has grasped learning to play the cello. Holding the beauty of the instrument in his own hand, Alex has found a love of music that has increased his love of life.

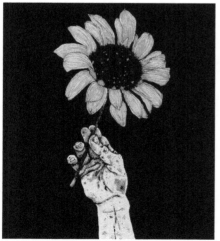

"Sunflower" by Josh Schwartz

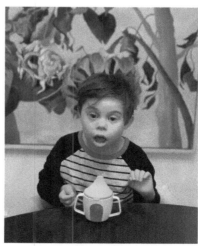

**Alex in front of "Wellbutrin"
by Elizabeth Castiglione**

But before a sunflower can bloom, its seed must be planted. It must be watered and showered in sunlight. Under these conditions, the flower thrives.

I believe that every child possesses the beauty and uniqueness of a flower. They all need nurturing, and that nurturing is different for daffodils than it may be for marigolds or roses, and so on. As an ELL Program Specialist, I work with K-7th graders, and I see it as my sacred responsibility to plant seeds, encourage with positivity, and help my students thrive. For me, teaching is not merely a job. It is a way of life. But I also know that, unlike flowers, people require a multitude of different gardeners if they are to bloom into the fullness and the beauty of themselves.

There is a wonderful Alexander den Heijer quote: "When a flower doesn't bloom, you fix the environment in which it grows, not the flower." It is April Beard who has planted the seeds of song within my youngest son, and our family is deeply indebted to her for all the ways she's enriched Alex's life. These in turn have enabled him to enrich the lives of others—even more.

A great teacher is a gift, and a blessing. They can see the unlimited potential in a seed and inspire it to bloom into the exact flower it was destined to be. A great teacher cultivates a diverse garden, cultivating the soil and bringing each unique bud of beauty into bloom. And, because of her work with Alex, every time I hear the song "Sunflower" from *Spider-Man: Into the Spider-Verse*, I think about how April Beard is a superhero teacher. Under her instruction, I have watched my third son, a child in whom other teachers might have failed to see unlimited potential, develop the superpower of being a person with Down Syndrome who is able to play the cello.

Looking back now, I think about how I, too, underestimated Alex's abilities. On the day of his first lesson, I didn't think he'd learn much and I suspected that, after a few weeks, April would give up, but it's been three years and Alex continues to improve and evolve and, more importantly, to love interacting with his instrument. That doubt about Alex's capacity wasn't the first time I underestimated him.

Moments after his birth, when I received my third son's diagnosis, I was devastated. It felt as if all my dreams for my youngest had just withered within me. I underestimated Alex. It wasn't long before those feelings evaporated. Now, I adore Alex. He's a gift and a blessing, and he keeps our family together. Whenever something gets hard, his love is like a rainbow after a storm. Brilliance emanates from him. He's not judgmental or sarcastic. His pureness is priceless.

At the same time, twelve years later, I've come to know that the world doesn't always view Alex the way I do. Some see his disability—the way Alex cannot talk, cannot walk, cannot feed himself, or use the facilities himself, and stay stuck there. When I think of all those things, my mind adds "yet." Alex cannot talk yet, cannot walk yet, etcetera. But the truth is that, whether or not he ever does those things, or hits any of the arbitrary "benchmark" expectations outsiders impose on him, I know that my son is already a sunflower. That doesn't mean that I don't notice the averted gazes when some of those we encounter see Alex, or the judgmental stares of those who ignorantly view him as a person taking up space and not contributing. I notice. And it hurts me, but not nearly as much as it limits them. Those who underestimate Alex miss out on the reality that he is someone capable, someone with gifts, someone that can shatter expectations—a person just like any other, and, at the same time, uniquely and exquisitely himself. And, every once in a while, I, too, underestimate my son. Each and every time I do, he outshines and exceeds all my expectations.

Alex has Trisomy 21, epilepsy, and hypotonia, but he is not Trisomy 21, epilepsy, and hypotonia. On the contrary, he is perfectly made and a gift, and I wouldn't change a thing about him. My sunflower son's language is his music. Through the playing of his cello is one of the ways—an audible way—that Alex speaks.

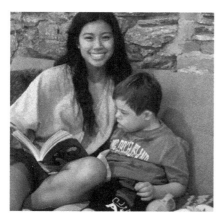

Hannah, a family friend, reading *The Phantom Tollbooth* by Norton Juster with Alex.

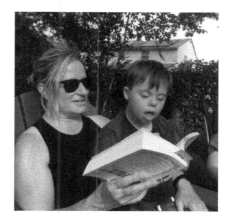

Alex and I reading *The Mysterious Benedict Society* by Trenton Lee Stewart.

In many ways, this book is April's and my song back to him. It is an invitation to listen to the music of his being. Along with the book, the two of us, aided by Jason Zeenkov, one of my best friend's son's and a "tech whiz," have painstakingly compiled and categorized video footage of many of Alex's cello lessons. You can find these lessons at www.upnotdownbook.com, and experience Alex experiencing music, which is a bit like watching a sunflower stretch upward and eastward in the direction of the sun.

I'm glad we have these videos. Through them, I can hold onto moments and memories. In the words of the poet, Robert Frost, "Nothing gold can stay." Alex has grown in his twelfth year to almost seventy pounds. And, over the twelve years since he's come into our lives, there have been many changes and challenges. We have lost loved ones. I have had breast cancer. My two oldest sons, Josh and Sam, have gone to college, a beautiful testament to their growth, and a bit of a heartbreak considering that their growing up means they almost never let me hug or kiss them anymore. They do, however, hug and kiss Alex. They play music with him, and each has their own unique bond with their baby brother.

No matter what, no matter the current life happening, or challenge, blessing, or obstacle, it is Alex who brings the music of our lives together to create a sweet symphony, along with my other sons Joshua and Sam. Sometimes, the song is off-beat. Other times, the instruments aren't always in tune. But, more often than not, I want to cry at the beauty of the orchestra.

Being Alex's parent, there are no solos. He requires accompaniment and, as a result of that, we've had the beautiful experience of surrounding ourselves with people who cherish, adore, guide him, and thereby make all of our lives better. Of course, my primary support and companion on this journey is Michael, my husband and Alex's father, and there are too many others to enumerate, but those that come immediately to mind are

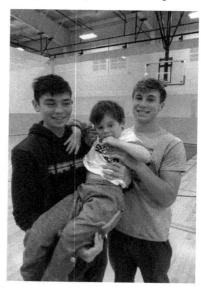

Josh, Sam and Alex at a S.N.A.P. (Special Needs Adaptive Program) soccer event.

Alex's extraordinary nurse, Nurse Tracy, his special education teacher, Megan Lindsay, speech therapist and eye gaze specialist, Barbara Davis, his physical therapist, Emma Mason (we love her, although Alex hates her for making him use his muscles), his occupational therapist, Kasey Brown, his previous special education teacher, Kim Gambone, and the personal care assistant, Kristen Culligan, who took the cover photo for this book and accompanied Alex to his first entire year of cello lessons. And, of course, there's April.

Alex:

I feel so special and blessed. I absolutely love my family. They do so much for me. I love the school I go to. My teachers and friends are the best. I love the world. Mom and Dad, even though I may not make you Mother's or Father's Day cards, or tell you how much I love you, I hope you know I do. I hope you know I think you are the best mom and dad in the whole wide world. Here, let me play a song for you.

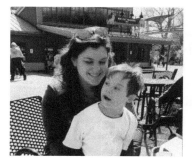

Alex and Kristen, his PCA (Personal Care Assistant) and now family friend.

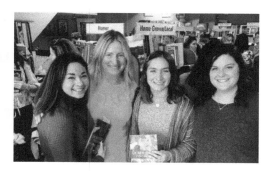

Kim Gambone, Megan Sabia, Kristen Culligan and Nancy at Nancy's book launch.

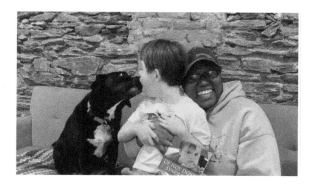

Alex and his home nurse, Tracy Seabrook with our dog, Jessica.

2 | April

At age 24, I landed my dream job. Since I was in seventh grade, I'd lived, breathed, and dreamed in the world of string playing, and since then my life trajectory had been shaped by my journey with music. I've had many meaningful experiences with music. Performing and teaching in beautiful places has inspired a true love of connecting children to the magic of music through playing an instrument. In retrospect, I can see that this love, connection, and musical magic is what the Schwartzes have brought into my life as an elementary school orchestra teacher.

I had finally reached my goal of teaching strings full time in a fantastic school district. I was to instruct third and fourth grade orchestra across five elementary schools, and I was thrilled that I would be doing exactly what I love to do in a big, diverse community. But perhaps most intriguing—and most nerve-wracking—was the prospect of creating an orchestra program at one of those schools in particular. Whereas the other elementary schools had long-established orchestra programs with already built community followings, one school was brand new. As the population of the area surged, the school district had added a fifth elementary school, and re-zoned and redistricted to create a beautiful new educational world. A panoply of amazing kids was coming together and I was going to be part of something new.

I felt like I could play a significant role in being able to build a new program within this newly-forming school community. The structure of this orchestra program was there for me to mold from the ground up, and that meant asking and answering never-before explored questions, like *What kind of program will this be?* And *Who will fill these sparkly new halls with mini violin renditions of Twinkle Twinkle Little Star?*

As I sorted through the instrument interest forms of sixty or so aspiring little musicians, I pictured a program like the one I went through as a ten-year-old at Branch Brook Elementary School on Long

Island. I pictured shuffling feet hurrying down the hallway to the music room, tiny instrument cases swinging in tiny hands, and students soaking up new information while I showed them simple yet essential techniques such as posture, plucking, and deciphering a new musical language.

I remembered the sparkly feeling of holding my viola for the first time, and the years that followed during which I came to realize the amazing gifts of music. For me, each and every instrument contains a reservoir of wisdom, and I was thrilled that I would be handing each child their instrument—and, with it, the potential for their own unexplored world of magic through music. When I began learning viola as a near fifth grader, I'd had no idea how my life would be sublimely shaped by my entry into the world of string instruments.

I started playing the viola the summer before fifth grade, taking a few introductory lessons from a local teacher with an instrument studio in her home. I can remember the smell of all the richly varnished, shining wood instruments hanging on every wall of her basement. My dad and I picked out my first viola there (although that memory is largely overshadowed by the teacher's two massive Samoyeds, more often mistaken as polar bears by my nine-year-old self, loafing about the room). Funnily enough, I had actually put down violin as my first choice of instrument on the form that came home with me from school. Viola was my second choice, clarinet third. I wonder if I'd been given my first or third choice if I would've still ended up engaged in this lifelong journey with stringed instruments, of which the viola has always been, and will always be, my favorite.

I don't particularly remember being any kind of extraordinary "practice-er" or performer when I started viola. In fact, I went through most of fifth grade and some of sixth grade feeling pretty nonchalant about my extracurricular playing time. I suppose, after the early seeds were planted, I required a few great teachers before my inner inspiration bloomed.

On my first day as an orchestra teacher, I couldn't help but remember the moment when I first wondered what it might be like to share the friendship and knowledge all secretly wrapped up in each instrument with students of my own.

I was in seventh grade, and my middle school orchestra teacher had a thoroughly embarrassing—but now in retrospect, brilliant and ultimately very meaningful to me—tradition of conducting your peers and friends in the orchestra on your birthday. The orchestra would play "Happy Birthday" while our teacher helped you wave your arms around in a three-beat conducting pattern, and you even got to hold the baton! If you were like me, you might stand on the podium glowing red, shoulders pushed up to your ears, trying to make yourself as small and unnoticeable as possible even though you were all your peers had to look at for the next eight measures of music. But surprisingly, after a few beats, I got caught up in the moment, and I didn't think about myself and how embarrassed I was. I instead thought about the students in front of me, making music with coordinated up bows and down bows—a sea of friends smiling, giggling and exchanging sideways glances to try to catch on to the notes. The music, or maybe the moment, or maybe both, washed over me. I don't think there was ever a moment after that where I didn't think I'd become an orchestra teacher. *What a sweet gig it would be,* I'd think.

Now that I'm living that dream, fourteen years later, I can say with certainty that it is a sweet gig!

When I began teaching orchestra to third and fourth graders, I had no idea the impact music education would have, not only on the students, but on me, too, because little did I know that the very first student to fill my beautiful new classroom with music—and hopes and dreams and brightness—would be fourth grader Alex Schwartz. Little did I know that this student in particular would bring to life the teaching philosophy I had believed in theory but had not yet had a chance to put into practice.

Before walking into the building on my first day of my new job, I reminded myself of the teaching philosophy I'd come up with as an assignment during my undergraduate degree: *Foster every child's connection to music as a dear and personal journey to them and celebrate every success along the way, no matter how small.*

Alex would breathe life into my theory of teaching as well as into a brand-new program—with every up bow, down bow, and every *pizzicato* in between.

3   **Nancy**

When I first started telling people, even well-meaning friends, "Alex is going to study the cello!" they reacted in one of two ways: Either they smiled and nodded in a way that conveyed the message *Poor, delusional Nancy, with her unrealistic dreams.* Or they said what they were thinking, "Umm... How is that possible?"

I have to admit that, even to me, playing the cello seemed about as likely for someone like Alex to accomplish as a flight to the moon. But I tried not to let my skepticism show. Even along the way, I was not without my doubts. When Alex started cello lessons and still could not take himself to the bathroom, there were moments when I thought *this is going to be impossible.*

It was April's unending belief in my son, her little cello student, that dispelled all these doubts—first mine, then others. Somehow, the rhythm of her teaching wiped away everyone's disbelief that Alex could achieve the unbelievable. And he has! Through April's example, I came to see yet again that, when we believe in ourselves and our path, anything is possible. *Anything.* This has been a continual lesson in my life, one in which, I'm afraid, I seem to suffer from situational amnesia.

That doesn't mean life is a smooth-ride, or that the path is always rainbows and sunbeams.

When the COVID-19 pandemic hit and lessons transferred to Zoom, I thought *We're doomed.* For weeks, I found myself feeling overwhelmed and inadequate. I tried to hold the cello, while encouraging Alex to sit up, and not drool, and hold the bow, and look at the music while simultaneously attempting to maneuver my laptop into the right angle so April could see Alex and give him feedback and encouragement. These times were not only difficult, they were exhausting! They made me ask, *why am I doing this?*—a question I asked of myself and of my husband, Michael, who encouraged me to stick with it.

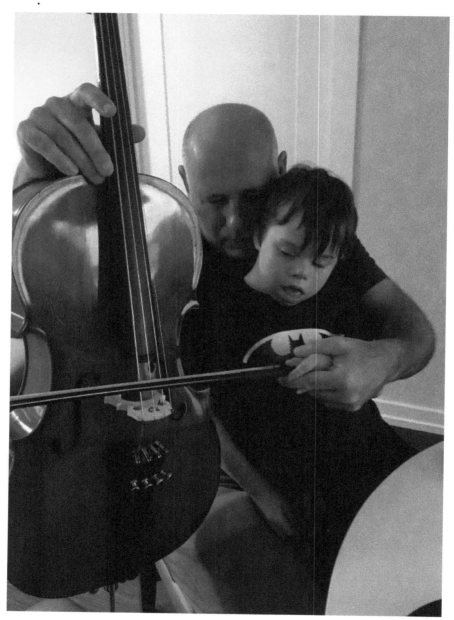

Alex and his dad play his new cello.

It wasn't until the day Alex's occupational therapist, Kasey Brown, sat in on the Zoom that she realized the problem—a problem that now seems so obvious "You need equipment to help hold the cello in place," she told me. "And you need to make sure Alex has a sturdy place to sit."

Kasey explained the basics of what I have since learned is called proximal stability, a strong grounded spot from which to use his body from a center of balance. She told me that Alex needed to be centered in himself and his position, and that his cello needed to be accessible if we had any hope of being successful on Zoom.

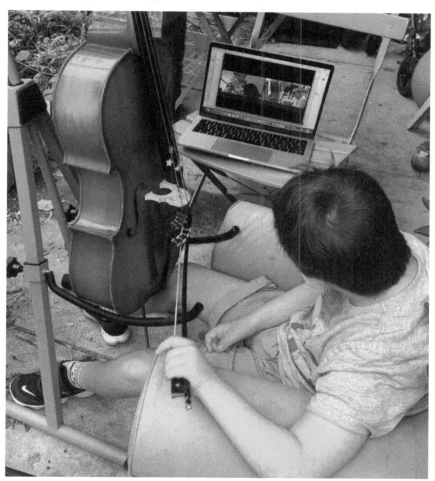

With help from a cello stand, and his feet planted on the ground, Alex plays his cello during a lesson over Zoom.

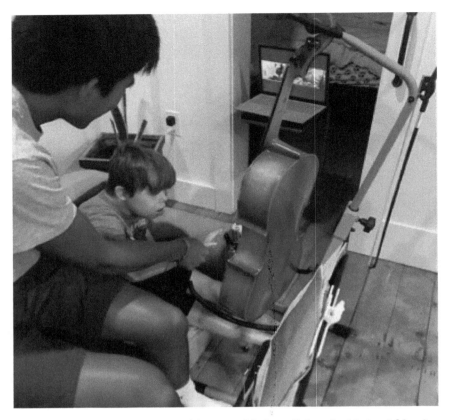

Alex during a virtual lesson with a guest helper, Dylan, Josh's best friend.

"But," she assured me, "with those modifications, it'll be a lot easier, and you'll both be a lot happier."

Her predictions have proved true. And, funnily enough, the implementation of proximal stability has become an enduring metaphor for what I strive to offer all my sons: a supportive foundation that enables them to flourish. And I'm so glad now that I didn't give up or decide to put Alex's musical explorations on hold until after we "got through" COVID.

Some may see Alex's lesson videos, hear him working on the same string with the same correlating color, and think *How mundane*. Yet, learning happens for him, and for so many others, through repetition. It is in the patience and persistence that he's embarked on a musical journey filled with hope. Hope for what he will be able to accomplish, personally, and hope that his example may inspire others to pursue their own seemingly out-of-reach accomplishments.

Alex's tenacity and his willingness to keep trying, keep learning, and keep growing, are a daily example to me. In his growth, I grow—and my heart grows. Sometimes, it expands so much it can't help but break a little.

As I'm writing this book, it has been a year since the world shut down due to the presence of a virus we cannot see, but which is threatening everyone everywhere. And, while it stops us from normalcy, the ordinariness of each day, of children attending school, of restaurants, discos, weddings, bar and bat mitzvahs, graduations, family gatherings, and friends, it has not stopped us from living. Or stopped others from dying.

During the span of the pandemic shutdown, Alex has lost his GaGa (his word for his grandma). It was not COVID-19 though, but an aggressive cancer. Eight months after her diagnosis, she was gone. This loss is impossible. The day of her funeral, we each put something in the box that would ease her soul's transition from here to the other side (and ease our hearts). Sam put a baseball in he'd caught during a Phillies game with Grandma and her fiancé, Allen (Allen, who was engaged to GaGa when she passed, has been a bonus PopPop to our family). Josh put a copy of his favorite Kurt Vonnegut book, *Slaughterhouse Five*. Michael left a piece of his art—a copper wire happy face—for his mom. I put in a red and white Valentine's Day doily from Alex. With help from his PCA (Personal Care Assistant Kristen, who has since become a family member and friend), my third son had lovingly printed his name on the doily. From myself, I put in an envelope that said *I love you* filled with Maxwell House coffee because we had spoken over coffee every morning for at least four or five years.

My morning coffees with GaGa were an indispensable part of my life and, even in her absence, I haven't stopped thinking about her every morning while I sip my Maxwell House. She was always so emotionally and spiritually supportive of all of us. In our chats, we talked about life, our family, and if Alex had had a good night the night before. Alex has nocturnal grand mal seizures, and, as a mother herself, GaGa could empathize with my sense of powerlessness in being unable to spare my son from pain. She'd lost a son, Michael's brother Barry, when he was 34, and I think the experience gave her a unique ability to savor her loved ones while they were living.

I know some people may not love—or even like—their mother-in-law. I loved mine so much that the sentiment is impossible to convey.

GaGa always made me feel like a daughter, as opposed to a daughter-in-law. She was there after my breast cancer surgery to remind me to be positive, when Alex was born to encourage me to see his light, and throughout all the ups and downs of marriage and motherhood. Sometimes, she and I conspired to get Michael to do things—like annual doctor's visits and the dreaded age-fifty colonoscopy. She felt like my friend, cheerleader and ally. Alex's too. Even today, when Alex swims at the gym with his brothers—Josh and Sam are lifeguards there—or his dad, I cry. GaGa was the first person I sent a photo of Alex swimming. She called me after receiving it to shout out her happiness. In fact, of all of us, she always cheered the loudest when a cello lesson video came from April. GaGa even made sure to get a gift for April at Christmas to show how much she appreciated the love and care April gave Alex.

My husband and I both wept during his speech for his mom at the service by her final resting spot. There were only ten of us, including the rabbi. Thanks pandemic. No shiva. No hugging. No standing in circles, reminiscing over Jewish soul food with those who knew and loved her. Michael's cousins, Mindy and Mark, did send food—bagels, lox and whitefish salad, olives and onions—and it was such a loving gesture that I cried when it came. But none of it felt sufficient to mourn GaGa's passing. Even had she not passed on during the pandemic, there'd have been no way to memorialize her that would have taken away our inner ache.

In his speech, I heard Michael say that his mom "never left him stranded" and I thought *that's right*. The love and devotion she gave us is unending. It continues even in her death. I still feel GaGa's presence and I know—we'll be okay. Sometimes, I can still feel GaGa cheering for Alex as he develops.

Alex is working on many things during his physical therapy, occupational therapy, and speech therapy. During PT, he works on sitting up, standing, and walking. All of this is challenging. He gets exhausted because of his severe hypotonia. Hypotonia—a state of low muscle tone—is common for many people with Trisomy 21. Uncommon, however, is playing the cello, which is strengthening Alex's body as well as his spirit.

Since GaGa's death, Alex's physical therapist, Emma, has suggested ways to use his wheelchair during his cello lesson, which have made it possible for Alex to hold the cello in the traditional way. Before that, he'd held the cello facing himself, but now he holds it facing outward.

Because of Emma's suggested modifications, Alex does not have to stabilize his body in space. The wheelchair gives him proximal stability—a way to stay stable without effort on his part. It also gives him license to concentrate on learning how to create music. In occupational therapy, Alex is working on his grasp, feeding himself, drinking independently, using the toilet, and more. Kasey, the occupational therapist who watched a cello lesson through Zoom then shared observations about how I could better support my son in supporting himself, has been an indispensable part of Alex's muscular and musical development.

After her insights, I bought a cello stand and she advised me to put something grippy on the bow to encourage Alex's capacity and stamina for holding it. April found us the exact right stand for Alex's physical requirements and re-introduced him to a grip-aiding tool for the bow called the CelloPhant™. She had used this tool with Alex during his first year of lessons for some time until she and Kristen felt it may have been too bulky or heavy, and potentially contributing to more grasp-fatigue. Now, two years later, Alex is stronger and has a wider hand span to more easily wrap around the CelloPhant™ and keep his grasp sustained. So even still, we continue to discover ways to adapt the cello so Alex can make beautiful music like any other sixth grader studying the cello. But music isn't the only area where Alex is finding new ways of expression and innovation.

Alex's speech therapist, Barbara Davis, made it possible to get an expensive computer with a program called Tobii Dynavox®, which is activated by eye-gaze technology. We climbed a mountain to get our medical insurance to help us provide this tool for Alex to learn to communicate. Barbara worked tirelessly, even though this was during the pandemic, when everything was even more difficult, to make the acquisition of Tobii Dynavox® possible for Alex. She came to our home—complete with mask and sanitizer—to instruct us on how to use the device, and how to teach Alex to use it.

If Alex looks at his desired statement and/or response, the technology speaks for him. His most common thing to say is "I am hungry." Recently, Barbara expressed amazement how Alex navigated through many menus and screens when she was across the room to get to the page on his Tobii that said, "I am hungry. I'll do it. I need help!" It is extremely difficult for Alex to learn how his thoughts can be translated through the gaze of his eyes, yet he is accomplishing this. He is expressing his thoughts more and more. At home, his brother Sam yelled downstairs, "Is Alex home?" "Yeah!" Alex screamed up clear as a bell.

Playing the cello translated into helping Alex sustain his grasp on a drinking cup, a crayon, a book, and toys. It is incredible that music has become one of his most useful and enduring forms of therapy and self-expression. It is motivating to Alex. When he hears a funky song on the radio, he will groove out to the beat. My friend, Marjorie, a musician herself, watched a video of Alex dancing to the song, "Funky Music Sho' Nuff Turns Me On," by Edwin Starr, and she told me, "That is what a true musician does. They feel the music."

Thanks to these cello lessons with April, Alex certainly feels the music.

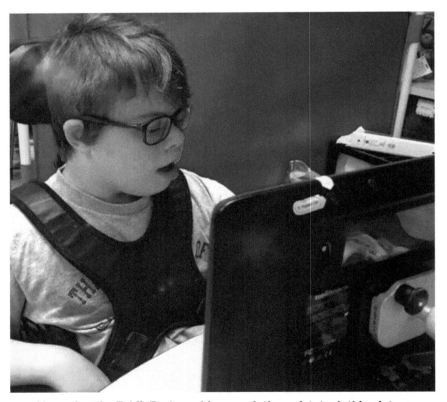

Alex using the Tobii. Barbara, his speech therapist, took this picture.

Alex:

I met Miss Beard today. She handed me the cello my mom and dad brought me for my birthday present. I love that she is going to teach me to play it. I enjoy music so much. I love when my mom or dad puts it on to lullaby me to sleep or play it when I start my day to fill me with hope for the new day. Miss Beard put the cello in my hand and showed me that I can use my hands to play it! Me!

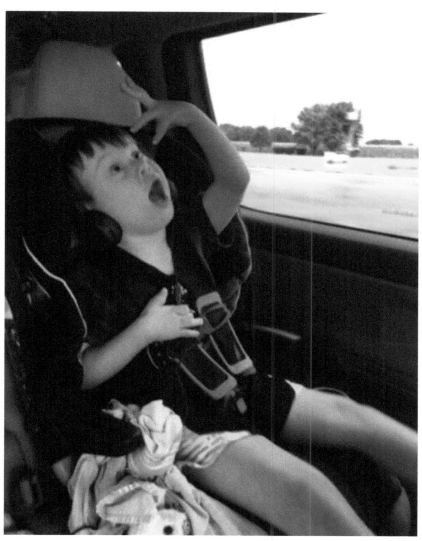

Alex grooving out to music on a long car trip to Virginia Beach.

4   April

I received Alex's interest form at the beginning of the year, along with many others. Alex's form indicated that he'd like to play the cello.

The instrument I was destined to play proved perfect for me, just as the cello has proved perfect for Alex. Having an instrument he can prop up and not have to hold up is essential, but I had no way of knowing that from Alex's simple form with its single check mark. All I knew was that the next step to get this new show on the road was to measure the children's arms for the correct sized instrument. All orchestral string instruments come in fractional sizes, and so measuring for the appropriate size is pivotal.

As I ascended to the fourth-grade hallway, my entire being was buzzing with excitement. This would be my first impression on the kids who would build this program, and I wanted them to see how much I already cared about their upcoming musical journey. The only other time I could remember being that expectant and full of possibility was after my middle school orchestra teacher suggested I take private lessons from a local teacher. I would end up studying with that private teacher all the way through senior year of high school, and she did so much—too much to comprehend sometimes—for me. She helped me prepare for solo competitions that allowed me to enter festival orchestras, for youth orchestra seating auditions and performances, and for college scholarship and entrance auditions. To me, she had the best job ever: teaching as an orchestra director in a public school district during the day, and then giving private lessons after school well into the evening. If she had inspired me so much and helped me get to all the places I could go, to think I could do that for kids from dawn to dusk too...

Playing the viola gave me a kind of voice, and I have come to believe that is true for Alex, too. It is so special to have that in common with him. I don't think I ever raised my hand once in high school. I was too shy, too self-conscious. If I had something important or of

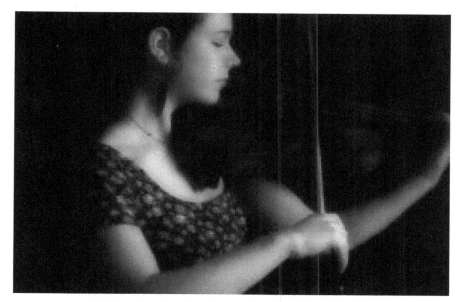

A high school era headshot of me playing my viola.

note to say, I'd be too scared at the prospect of my answer being "wrong" to even attempt to answer, but in the colorfully painted hallway of my high school designated as the "Music Suite," it was a different story. Around my high school orchestra teacher, Mr. C, I could talk for hours and be myself. I could act silly with my friends in orchestra class, maybe even call out an answer or two. I would demonstrate on my instrument, stand up secretly proud when Mr. C would acknowledge me for performing in some honorary orchestra or for receiving a high performance rating.

Now that I am a public school orchestra teacher, I get to be on the other side of this; I get to support students in their love for music and to see them be acknowledged for their hard work in a skill that takes a lot of, well…hard work. I see the students who, like me, need to summon a lot of courage just to raise their hand, and those same students who, like me, can't help but to smile at the satisfying feeling of drawing a bow across the strings of their instrument.

I wasn't daunted by the prospect of hard work when I had my first chance to pursue my one and only career dream. I was ecstatic. I went into each fourth-grade classroom and called out the names of the students on the interest forms so they could come out in the hallway for measuring.

But when I called Alex's name, he wasn't there.

"Oh!" the classroom teacher said, "Alex is in Ms. Gambone's room." I made a note to find him later. However, by the time I'd finished measuring the long line of other children, I saw Alex's Personal Care Assistant, Kristen, smiling warmly as she pushed a boy in a wheelchair down the hallway towards me.

"Alex, this is Ms. Beard," Kristen said. "Ms. Beard, this is Alex."

I learned in that moment that Alex was a soon-to-be cellist with Trisomy 21, also known as Down syndrome. As Alex and I looked at each other, I noticed his bright brown eyes were full of expression. *Now here's a student with potential. Here's a student where we are going to celebrate every inch of progress and every success, no matter how small. Here's a student who's going to define what this music program is all about.*

5   **Nancy**

When I was three years old, my parents enrolled me in ballet class with a teacher named Miss Bianca at Abington Art Center.

Miss Bianca was a strict ballet teacher. She yelled at me when I stood on my tippy toes at the barre. I loved seeing my form in the mirror and standing on my tippy toes reminded me of the beautiful ballerinas I got to see dance in *The Nutcracker* by the Pennsylvania Ballet (now known as the Philadelphia Ballet). And, when I wore my bathing suit to class because it had a little skirt like a tutu, she shook her head, clearly conveying her disapproval. We all held the barre as she explained, first put your feet in first position, demi-plié, second position demi-plié, third position, fourth position, and fifth position. I loved putting my feet in fifth position. Okay, repeat with grand-plié. She counted. We followed her directions, scared of her correction if we missed a beat. Miss Bianca said, "Come to the floor," which meant we would be dancing in front of the mirror. That was my favorite! I learned the technical terms and the techniques Miss Bianca shared. She was full of poise, love, grace, and discipline.

In college, I minored in dance at Temple University. Dancing in African dance, modern and ballet gave me a love for dance that is still in my heart.

After ballet came piano lessons with Mrs. Goldhersh, in her home with her four cats as our audience. In addition to her many cats and baby grand piano, Mrs. Goldhersh had stacks of sheet music and a wide, inviting smile. Every time I went to her home to study piano with her, I brought a small bag with our notebook, and my own, simple sheet music. Mrs. Goldhersh explained the keyboard and notes. She taught me to read music and how to play scales on the piano. The scent of cats permeated the lesson, but the love Mrs. Goldhersh had for music and conveying how to play it to me made the cat smell disappear (almost). I did not love to practice, but I loved my lessons. Occasionally, a cat would jump on her piano to help teach me. I loved how my

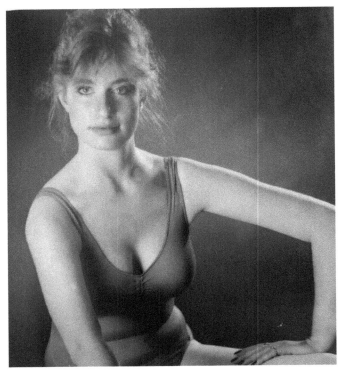

A ballet portrait of Nancy in high school.

mom would be so happy when I played this one song in my book. It was rhythmic and graceful like the ballet I learned. I had a joy when I could read the music and play what it said, and I knew that this would be a skill I would always enjoy. I loved learning to play Beethoven's *Für Elise*. I stopped playing with Mrs. Goldhersh when my parents divorced and we moved from Cheltenham to Northeast Philadelphia. There I had a new piano teacher, Mr. Liebskin. He came to the apartment where my mom and I lived, along with our upright piano—a reminder from our old home. Mr. Liebskin focused on pop songs rather than on classical. He wrote the letters under the notes so I did not have to read the music.

And then came violin lessons with Mrs. Curner, who was an amazing violinist. She had a passion for the violin and shared it with me at the Settlement Music School in Jenkintown, and sometimes at her home. She taught me to hold the violin under my chin, to use good posture when holding the violin and holding the bow. Mrs. Curner taught me the names of the strings and shared the names of some amazing violinists with me. I loved my time with her and how she taught me to use rosin on the bow. She said I was a natural violinist. Mrs. Curner pointed out that I had the perfect padding on the underside of my fingers for playing on the strings. She made me feel smart and capable each time we met, much like the way April makes Alex feel each cello lesson by focusing on what he can do, not what he cannot, yet. Mrs. Curner's daughter gave me a tiny bottle of colored sand from a beach in Israel. I still have it.

Again, I did not love the practicing part. My mom, the artist, always creating fun and interesting things for me, made me a tiny black velvet cushion from a pretty evening gown so that I could keep the violin at the right level while also keeping my chin comforted from the wood base of the violin. Once, she took my soft plaid shirt I had outgrown and made the pockets into little stuffed animals she called, "Pattie Plaids." Mom liked to make up nicknames. Another time she sewed lips and lipsticks, with fabric compacts made from silver and hot pink silk for my friend Susan's sweet sixteen. She designed cartoons, like the New Yorker, as well as greeting cards. When I was in elementary school, she took empty octagon glass bottles and filled them with light blue Epsom Salt scented lavender for my teachers' gifts.

The violin became a small piece of my heart and of my life, and although I'd never have guessed it at the time, I have come to believe that G-d was crafting me to learn music, and especially string instruments, so that I would have the skills—limited and rusty though they may be—to support Alex and Josh (Sam never really took to instruments) in their musical journeys. G-d, aided by my parents.

My dad and mom made certain that I listened to Mozart piano sonatas, the Bach *Cello Suites*, Shuly Natan, and more. I'll always remember Dad moving his hands through the air to conduct as we listened. Family friends, Esta, Eli, Sam, and Robbie, took me to an Itzhak Perlman concert when I was studying that year. I recall sleeping in my chair for most of the performance. As the lights came back on in the concert hall, my eyes blinked open, and I remember leaving the hall relaxed and peaceful, but I did not realize the genius I was fortunate to hear.

When I named my violin "Amy" (Mrs. Curner said every instrument deserves a name), my teacher asked if I knew what "Amy" meant in French?

"No," I said.

She told me it means "friend" (*ami*). May Alex always have human friends, and his cello. Alex has named his cello, which he emphatically informed me is a girl, "Geri," which means "rules with a spear." Alex appreciates beautiful ferocity.

He also appreciates classical composers. Our favorite song to listen to together is Bach Cello Suite No. 1 in G Major, but Alex's musical tastes are eclectic and wide-ranging. He enjoys everything from Mozart to The Weekend, and he especially loves to groove out to funk music. Because of his studies with April, he has come to find his own inspiration. Because of who he is inside, maybe partly because of the musical traits he inherited from me, he feels the music like a true musician.

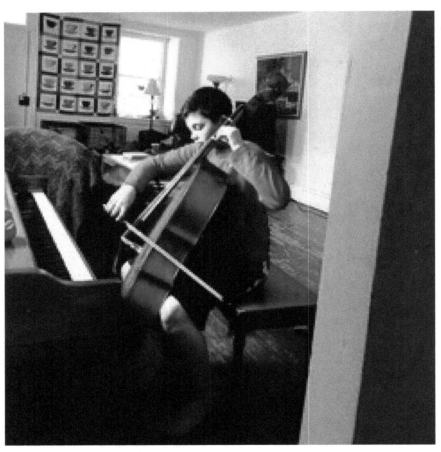

Nancy's oldest son, Josh, practicing the cello.

Alex:

Thank you, Ms. Beard, for knowing I can. I can learn new information about music, and the cello. Thank you for treating me like a brilliant student, for catching the positive things I learn, and for believing in me. I am blessed to have a cello teacher like you. I am grateful for your courage, and the gift of your teaching. I love how you accept me. You create a brave space for me to grow, and, in doing so, you show the world what is possible through belief in ourselves and in others.

6 April

After measuring Alex's arm, I let my pen hover over the sizing form I'd be sending home with him. I was debating between a half-size and a quarter-size cello. *He's not quite big enough for a half-size, but will the quarter-size require too much fine motor coordination? Will the half-size be better for macro-movements and allow for him to hear more resonant sound? And the wheelchair...*

I was concerned that parts of the wheelchair might get in his way or interfere with the positioning of the instrument.

Could he sit without it? Could the armrests on it fold down so he can move his arms horizontally? Could the footrests move so we could get the cello centered in front of his body?

Quarter-size, I decided, and wrote the fraction on the form. An instrument that's too big can be discouraging, and even cause injury. A smaller cello would be safer, and why not think long-term and promote more fine motor coordination growth and practice through music?

I'm so grateful, in retrospect, that I took the time to think through the size of Alex's cello. Three years in, he's not ready for a bigger cello yet and, in seeing how Alex interacts with his instrument, I can tell that its size allows him to maneuver physically as well as musically.

From the moment we met, I was so excited to be working with Alex. At the same time, the world can erect roadblocks and barriers for non-typical learners, and I knew that we were likely to encounter speedbumps.

I am beyond grateful to have been raised by people who are the best problem solvers I've ever met. My PopPop is an ingenious inventor, creator, and fixer-upper, and my wise mom and handy dad each react to obstacles with calmness, evaluating their choices before taking decisive action.

Alex was *not* and is *not* a problem. The world is simply logistically easier to navigate for some people than for others. Having been conditioned to meet challenges head-on came in handy as I thought about how best to maximize Alex's learning, and how to modify my teaching to give him what he needed, when he needed it.

One speedbump was scheduling. I was only in the elementary school Alex attended one and half days a week to teach between 70 and 80 third and fourth graders. This was not uncommon for an orchestra teacher, as many often teach multiple grade levels in multiple buildings and, although we do generally combine students into learning cohorts, more often than not, we find ourselves needing to become logistical acrobats.

There were certain periods in the children's schedules when I could not pull them out for lessons. In addition, I wanted to have separate groups for violins, violas, and cellos, and I didn't want the lesson group sizes to be so big that students wouldn't be able to get the moments of individualized attention required when learning an instrument. The lesson periods were only thirty minutes; however, realistically, by the time the students came down to the orchestra room, unpacked, tuned, and asked for materials or repairs to their instruments, I would be lucky to get in twenty minutes of content.

As much as I wanted Alex to be a part of the program and a part of the orchestra, I wouldn't have felt right putting him in a lesson group with other children. I wanted my full attention to be with Alex, as his short-term and long-term musical goals would be different from the other children's, and the way his instrument would need to be supported would be more hands-on. Of course, Alex would still learn all the fancy technical musical terms in Italian, like all my other students. He'd still listen and play along to the great works of Mozart and Beethoven. He'd still watch the cello greats Yo-Yo Ma and Jacqueline du Pré perform a varied repertoire, and we'd still observe their techniques and emulate them together. We'd fiddle, we'd focus, we'd discover music much the same as every other string group I'd have, but the process would be different. The inner workings would be differentiated, but the outcome would be just as beautiful. I decided I'd fit Alex in wherever I could—maybe during part of my lunch, or in one of the two 20-minute prep periods at the beginning of the day, or at the very end of the day before our 3:30 dismissal, or some combination of the above. *Okay*, I thought. *One-on-one sessions and scheduling will be easy fixes.*

The other "problem," which was more overwhelming, pervasive, and bewildering at times—and a problem I still struggle with today, although to a lesser extent—had to do with my training and conditioning. There is pressure amidst classical music traditions of learning and teaching string instruments in a somewhat prescriptive, set way. As a classically trained musician myself, I very much value teaching classical and traditional elements like correct posture (how one holds the instrument), and note reading practices based on centuries-old music notation. What would other music educators think if I taught Alex a "non-traditional" way of playing the cello? An adapted way that spun everything around and turned music on its head to make it accessible for his unique needs and abilities? What would Alex's parents think? How could I set him up to be the most successful on his instrument—to get the most out of his experience—while still falling under this "classically trained musician" umbrella?

I worried a lot about not being fair to Alex if I didn't teach him the way I'd been trained to teach. But then I worried a lot that if I did teach him the way I was taught, I still wouldn't be fair to him.

I'd experience waves of "imposter syndrome" and many moments of self-doubt. But each time those feelings would arise, I'd remind myself of a foundational teaching philosophy that has rooted me back to myself and my love of music and teaching, and back to how I needed to think in order to be the teacher Alex needs me to be.

One of the most important things I learned from my studies with my graduate school viola professor is that music needs a vehicle to flow through. We must set ourselves up to be a natural channel for the instrument to sing and for the music to flow. My teacher's many passionate and inspiring outpourings on this subject rang through me as I reminded myself to focus on what being an educator is really about: *it's about Alex, it's his journey.*

Less than 24 hours after I finished filling out the cello size and rental form, and handed it to Kristen, I received this email:

> Hi Ms. Beard,
>
> I am thrilled that Alex will get a chance to try the cello. Will lessons I hope be during the school day?
>
> Have a great day!!
>
> Thank you,
> Nancy

I replied.

> Good morning!
>
> Thank you so much for getting in touch! I'm so glad Alex will be playing the cello! I'm looking forward to working with him. Yes, lessons are during the school day. The lesson times

rotate; however, I am wondering if he'd like to come at a more permanent time each week so that we can work one-on-one. Is this something you think would work in his schedule, even if it's just 20 or so minutes in the afternoon that he might have free? I am in the building Mondays all day and Tuesday mornings. I am definitely free from arrival to 9:15 and from 3:10 to dismissal, if that is an option for him as well. If not, I can build around whatever time could work for him.

Thank you!

Musically,

April Beard

Nancy and I soon began a regular, weekly correspondence. We wrote about music, about Alex, about ways we could innovate and collaborate. I quickly discovered that she is not only a wonderful mother, but an experienced and passionate educator herself who understands that above all, there is a great need for, and value in, setting every student up for the success they deserve to experience and own. Nancy was—and is, and has always been—wonderfully willing to accommodate my requests. As we flowed, the music began to flow—for Alex and through Alex.

At our first lesson, Alex and Kristen came into the orchestra room at the end of the school day. I was nervous as I asked, "Could Alex possibly sit in a chair instead of in his wheelchair?"

I didn't want to make him feel uncomfortable during a new experience for him, but Kristen easily plopped him down into a classroom chair. Alex sat up beautifully, looking around the room. I took out his mini-cello (that might've actually been the first time I held a cello that small!), and pulled the endpin out. As I started to bring the instrument near him, his eyes filled with wonder and curiosity. Alex beamed. I beamed. Kristen beamed.

I strummed the strings, and the whole room felt warm and sparkly — a feeling I get every time I see this transfer of happiness happen through music. Handing a student their instrument for the first time gives me a lot of joy. It's like the feeling you get when giving someone a really special gift.

For our initial, exploratory lesson, I set Alex up in the traditional way, with the back of the cello resting on his sternum and his knees on either side of the cello. He was able to reach around, with some help, to strum across the strings on the front of the cello, but he kept pulling his arms back to his sides very quickly. Alex had this same tendency to

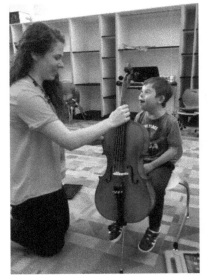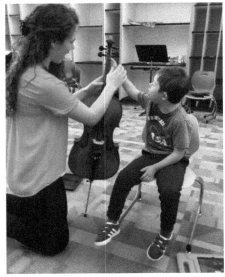

These photos were taken during Alex's first cello lesson. Kristen took these photos, and his face says it all. He was curious and sat up tall and proud in a chair, and the rest is history!

withdraw his arms back into himself for much of our early work together, but we were able to grow his capacity to reach and extend. In fact, over the next year, he improved greatly with this. Now, he's got a swimmer's reach that enables him to fully stretch.

Personally, I found it challenging to support the cello and Alex at the same time. I knew the motions I wanted him to make, but I couldn't get the cello to stay supported in its usual setup like this. I felt like I needed another set of arms. Yes, Alex would eventually be this other set of arms after gaining some strength and familiarity with the instrument. He wasn't there yet and my musical intuition told me that if I didn't find a way to innovate, we'd both get frustrated and I wouldn't be able to inspire him to stay with the cello long enough to learn how to support the instrument on his own.

So, I turned the cello around (insert classical musicians gasping here). With no real plan or intention of keeping this setup in the long-run, I felt it was more of a creative work-around to initiate some progress, as the learning had stalled with the cello the other way, the "right" way. With this being an antithetical way to my classical training, I told myself it was a temporary modification, as I found myself kneeling on the floor, holding the cello forward (but in classical reality, completely backward!) to Alex. It seemed that it was only this way that I could encourage Alex to reach out for the cello and maintain eye contact with the strings so he could see just how the instrument worked and made sounds. I wanted him to realize the cause and effect, saying to him, "*You*, Alex, can be the driver—the architect—of all the rich and rewarding sounds that this thing can make." And, despite my initial fear—the *Oh no! What have I just done?* moment inside me—Alex lit up. He reached out to the cello and it almost seemed as if the cello reached back out to him.

I remember feeling a great relief that Alex enjoyed his first lesson, and even in our short twenty minutes together, his positive energy, focus, and joy around the cello made me feel confident that Alex was going to be successful with this. Still, I remained less confident in myself. After all, it was only the third week of school, my first official week of teaching.

7 Nancy

One of my great inspirations since even before Alex's birth, but especially over the last twelve years, has been Dr. Sharon M. Ravitch, Professor of Practice at the University of Pennsylvania's Graduate School of Education.

Sharon and I went to Akiba High School together. She was a year younger, but I was—and am—friends with her older sister, Liz, and so Sharon and I always liked each other a lot and were friendly, but from afar.

Dr. Ravitch is a distinguished Teaching, Learning, and Leadership Division Principal Investigator, Semillas Digitales Initiative Fulbright Fellow, 2021-2022 GIAN Scholar Government of India, 2018-present Creator, and Flux Pedagogy. Her credentials are more than a little intimidating. And, yet, her advice has always been entirely accessible. Partly due to my admiration for her work, partly because of our tenuous yet enduring connection, I was fortunate enough to be able to attend her Flux Pedagogy: Transformative Leadership in Times of In-equity Institute, through Penn GSE, and to hear her speak about how we need to develop a "radical growth mindset." I love the concept of a "radical growth mindset." It feels like without having been able to name it before Dr. Ravitch gifted me with the terminology, April, Alex, and I have used our own radical growth mindsets to support and amplify our ability to accomplish all we have, individually and collectively. Each time we set out to do some new thing, or understand a new concept, we decided "yes—this will be possible," and we're always right, whether immediately or eventually.

In addition to radical growth mindset, through Dr. Ravitch's institute I learned about radical compassion, another key element that has supported and sustained me. As my lifelong idol explained, radical compassion extends to others and it also extends to ourselves. Having understanding for myself, my limits and my needs, is something I have begun to practice daily. Despite what I'd previously believed, radical self-care isn't necessarily mud masks, pedicures, and spa retreats—although those can be fabulous ways to cultivate self-care. Radical self-care can be taking a break, or figuring out what will make my heart feel right. It is the skill of stepping back, and seeing myself at a soul level. It is doing what I need to remain on the path of what matters most to me.

What matters most to me are relationships. I see my role in this world as to give as much as I can to others while also giving to myself. As a mother, this can feel like a daily, almost meditative practice.

Okay, Nancy, bring your focus back to you. C'mon, Nancy, pay attention to the moment.

I think music has helped me to be more compassionate to myself and to others. Not just Alex's music, but our family's history of and enduring love for music. It's like coming home.

Josh, my first son, chose to play the cello in fourth grade. His teacher was a kind music teacher at his school, Roberts Elementary School. It made me happy that he chose the instrument his dad had

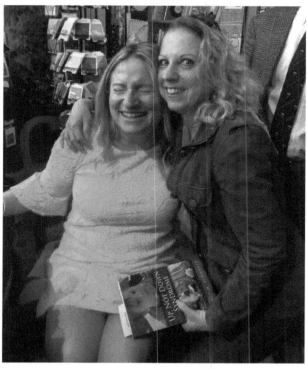

Nancy and her sister-in-law, Sheryl, at the book launch for my first book.

bought me when I was pregnant with him. I'm not sure if it was coincidence or kismet. All I know is that, when Josh was still in utero, I saw this extraordinary cello in our local music shop's window. Michael bought it while we were on a stroll in the town of Wayne, Pennsylvania. He wanted me to have a gift for carrying his son. It's funny, with our second son, he bought me a vanilla latte from the Gryphon Café, and a bouquet of flowers from our garden. When Alex was born he bought a pale blue satin-footed bear for Alex. And, of course, the true gift is the love we have for our babies. Love is all we need, and want. Well, not all. I always wanted to play the cello because of the beauty of its sound, the soulful way it spoke to me. I had lessons from my colleague, Robyn Gold, in the Downingtown Area School District. Robyn was patient with me trying to learn the strings, the placement of my fingers, and the new notes they made. Learning up bow from down bow seemed impossible to me at the time, but Robyn would calmly re-explain how to make the bow move and where to place it. I learned to read the notes and play "Twinkle Twinkle Little Star" and it's variations in *Suzuki Cello School, Volume 1*.

In retrospect, I was forced to modify my playing around the needs of my pregnant body just as Alex has been required to modify his positioning and playing in ways that enable him to grace the world with his music. I loved playing for Josh. I loved Michael for giving me the gift of an untapped reservoir of musical possibilities, as well as the gift of our first son.

Josh came into the world and my cello took a rest as I learned about being a mom. Years later in elementary school, Josh had a concert and my heart filled with pride as I watched him play on stage, the notes carrying beauty. He broke my heart the next year when he, and his friend, Ryan, decided to play the trombone, leaving his cello to be returned to the store where we'd rented it from in West Chester, Pennsylvania. Still, I was proud he'd tried the cello. I hope someday he will return to it.

Sam, our second son, was born sixteen months after Josh. I was now a mom of two. As Sam grew, I missed my cello. I found through a colleague in my school building a new cello teacher in the area, Jie Jin, who is from Shanghai, China. Her playing is gorgeous. She made the cello seem as beautiful as ever to me. Jie taught me, and I loved it. I loved it so much that I wanted Josh and Sam to take lessons from her, but Jie explained that Josh and Sam should start with learning notes on the piano before studying a string instrument.

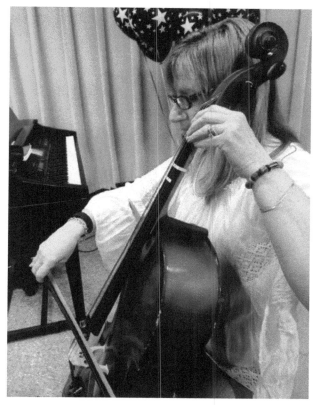

Nancy playing the cello with the Wayne Elementary School Orchestra.

Sam tried piano lessons with Jie. He came home with the letters of the notes written in eyeliner on the knuckles of his hand and cried that he hated the piano. He stopped while Josh continued.

We never know which teachers, or which loves, will resonate, or how they'll resonate, or how our influence can shape those we are closest to. Josh still loves the piano and Sam, who loves music, is a passionate and gifted soccer player. Alex is my little cellist.

April and her powerful teaching, her unwavering belief in Alex, regardless of his challenges, physical or otherwise, have shaped my youngest son's daily life and have enriched the lives of our family. Sometimes, I'll be moving a load of laundry from the washer to the dryer, taking a walk, or hugging Alex, and I'll think, *What would life be like if we hadn't met April?*

It's a thought that sends shivers down my spine. Then, I'll bask in the reality that April is a part of our lives, and that the cello is a part of Alex's life. And I'll recall my own long-ago violin days with Mrs.

Curner and be reminded, yet again, of a gifted educator's ability to have a positive influence. And of my more recent teachers and the growth they've brought into my life, musically and otherwise. Once discovered, music has the power to evoke magic. But that power can be elusive. For Alex to discover it required an outstanding educator. For Alex to become the musician that he is, he needed April.

Alex:

Me? I get to play this beautiful cello? You think I can do it? You believe in me? I get a chance to show what I can learn? Thank you. I am amazing. I won't let you down. Watch what I can do. Look Mom; I will make you proud.

8 | April

On my first designated day to work with Alex, I wasn't sure how he would react to learning the cello. The whole thing felt like an unknown, and I wanted it to be a positive experience for him and wanted to be able to engage him. My hope was that he'd like it and he'd take some sort of initiation with the cello.

Now that I knew he'd liked our first lesson, I wanted to keep the momentum going. Alex was in my schedule each week at the end of the day at 3:10, so Kristen would bring him down and we'd work until about 3:30 when it was time for him to take the bus home. Kristen proved to be an enormous support during his lessons and an indispensable part of me building a rapport with Alex. She'd lift him from his wheelchair and kneel beside him with me. She helped me recognize what he was communicating, and she'd tell me about his day and keep him engaged with prompts by echoing things I said, asking encouraging questions, and praising him. She was his cheerleader, celebrating his successes, no matter how small, because she knew Alex much better than I did, and I fed off of her cues and learned through her example, ways that Alex preferred to relate. Kristen's help showed me how to be who Alex needed me to be.

Although I'd decided pretty soon into his first lesson that, against all classical traditions, we should continue with the cello spun around to face Alex, I still had my doubts about how long this technique should last. I knew that, eventually, I'd work with Alex to transition the instrument to face outward, but I willed myself to allow it to be okay that for the time being, Alex was going to do things his own way. Seeing Alex light up with love for the cello dispelled my fears about whether or not the technique was right for him, but I had some insecurities about what Nancy would think. In one of our early email exchanges, she'd mentioned having her own experiences with the cello, as well as the violin and the piano, and I worried that she might judge me for teaching her son in a way that defied all the rules.

Any classically trained musician would feel an internal wince on seeing my non-traditional cello set up with Alex, and part of me felt that way too, but I reminded myself of the philosophy I'd carefully and lovingly crafted as an undergraduate student, looking forward to a future I could only hope would come to me. My job was and is to set Alex up to be as successful as he could be on this instrument. This was *his* journey of becoming a musician, and the doors were, and still are, wide open for him to enter into and become his own musician.

By having the cello face Alex, he was able to establish and build upon these skills:

- **Eye contact:** Alex could see the strings as they vibrate. He could see me and my reactions as he listened to my instructions. And, perhaps very importantly, he could see out to whoever was watching (whether his aide, or Nancy, or any other audience member). It seemed to be that, as Alex notices himself being positively recognized, he glows with pride.

- **Tracking:** he could watch his hand move horizontally as we did exercises like "bear claw" strums across the four strings to work on strengthening his three rows of knuckles. He could watch his fingers as we plucked across each string individually. He could watch the bow as he moved it back and forth and from string to string.

- **Engagement and initiative:** keeping the instrument squarely in front of him helped Alex to stay engaged while keeping the cello available and accessible for when he wanted to initiate movement without my help.

- **Arm extension:** this is a big one! Reaching out toward the cello had become a main focus with his skill development, and has ended up serving him both in playing the cello and in the acquisition of other activities of daily living skills.

For about two years, we kept the cello facing Alex. When we were in person, the back of the cello would lean against me, and I'd support the body of the cello with my own body so that I had two free arms to reach around and help guide Alex.

Alex is very strong at showcasing skills in his own ways, both within the course of our lessons and outside of our lessons—in the other areas of his life. Specifically, from our first session onwards, Alex has been applying what he learns through music in other settings.

Early on in our work together, Alex was reluctant to outstretch his arms, and a lot of prompting was needed to get him to reach for the cello. Now, he rarely has any reluctance at all. Since beginning our cello lessons, Alex's shoulders and arms stemming from his pectoral muscles have become much stronger and more pliable.

We humans are symbiotic, and it is through what Nancy sometimes refers to as the "village approach" that Alex has come to flourish. I think the many extracurricular experiences Nancy gives Alex, like swimming lessons each week, have helped immensely with his cello learning as well as his confidence. Maybe it's not any one thing. Maybe his experiences playing cello have translated into his aptitude in the pool, and his experiences swimming have helped him to become a more independent cellist.

Alex is always outperforming his previous self, always learning and growing and (quite literally) stretching beyond his prior capacity. By being patient but persistent in showing him that arm extensions are a pivotal movement, I was able to help him see that cause and effect. I think he'd come to realize: *I can't make a sound without reaching forward.*

Once Alex began his swimming lessons, we were able to relate the two activities to each other, and eventually arm mobility and extension became a strength of Alex's.

"Use your swim stroke," I'd tell him, and he'd reach to pluck or bow. "Swim, swim, swim!"

A huge touchstone in the teaching philosophy I believe in is *connecting*. I try to show my string students that playing an instrument can be connected to anything in the world, and vice versa. Music is math, physics, history, grammar, physical education, psychology, geometry, and so many other things beyond that. Connecting is everything in my lessons.

I remember one of my fourth-grade violinists exclaiming mid-lesson, "Wow! Music makes so much sense when you relate it to other things in the world!" I loved her "aha!" moment. That single sentence—*music makes so much sense when you relate it to other things in the world*—is everything I want my students to realize, and the other way around, too: the world makes so much sense when you relate it to music.

Like his peers, and like all of us, Alex is discovering more and more of the world each day. And one of my greatest joys in working with him is seeing how music has become one of his paths to connecting to and relating to his external and internal experiences.

I knew from the moment I broke with my classical music ranks and redirected the instrument to face him that Alex would teach me to become a better connector. And that has proved to be true, both inside and outside of the classroom.

I'm the type of person who always cares what people think. I'm a people pleaser, so in a way, going against classical tradition, saying "this is what's best for Alex, and best for me as his teacher," revealed to me that this is what it feels like to experience all those educational buzzwords that were in my music education textbooks, words like: *flexibility, adapting, accommodations.*

Throughout my work with Alex, and my other students, I hope to connect as many sensory experiences with the instrument as possible, and to foster a sense of curiosity and exploration. At the Crane School of Music, my violin techniques and string education professor and adviser, Dr. Hertz, taught me that so much more resonant learning can happen and truly stick when students discover something seemingly on their own, while the teacher quietly scaffolds, waiting behind the scenes, for that beautiful student-led moment of unearthing.

To face the cello strings toward Alex opened up opportunities for him to make his own discoveries. But there have been so many moments beyond that when I've had to find different ways of conveying concepts and different ways of inspiring Alex to explore.

Working with burgeoning musicians whose ways of learning aren't typical have inspired me to try to find little ways to help him connect. For instance, Alex communicates in nonverbal ways, his body acts as his voice and he takes things in through his physical experiences in ways that are palpable yet which he can't convey in words yet, as Nancy would say, and I've come to say, too. When I realized Alex's attunement to stimuli, one of the first thoughts I had was to let the cello make contact with his shins. Knowing that each string has its own vibration frequencies, I suspected that the feel of these vibrations could aid in the way Alex understands and interprets pitch. The highest string on the cello, the A string, vibrates more quickly and with more tension. The lowest string, the C string, vibrates more slowly and with a looser feel.

I often wonder about Alex's perception of pitch and look for communication from him to see if he's developing his internal ear. Alex is very expressive in his face and eyes, and that has become an effective mode of communication for us. When he's happy, his eyes squint up, and when he's alert, his eyebrows raise up a little. When he's really focused on his task, he leans toward the cello, getting his eyes as close as he can to the strings. When he hears something intriguing, he looks at me, Nancy, or Kristen, with a question in his gaze. I try to return his expressiveness with my own animation, hoping to confirm exactly what he's sensing.

One of my favorite activities and learning experiences with Alex has been working on "down bows" and "up bows." In cello playing, a down bow is when a cellist pulls the bow across the strings to the right, while an up bow is a push in the opposite direction. After a few lessons working on this, I asked Alex to show me a down bow and to show me an up bow, which he did—with his eyes and head! I was delighted! I don't think there is a better feeling than being inspired by your student's responses. I was expecting him to give a little nudge one way or another with his arm or hand, but instead on that day, he swung his eyes and gently leaned his head to the right and left in a way that mimicked the gliding path of the bow. I followed his lead, and even today Alex often demonstrates his skill in this way when I say, "Show me an up bow! Show me a down bow!" After Nancy published her first book about Alex, *Up, Not Down Syndrome*, I would find it so funny that Alex seems to have preference for up bows, frequently initiating repetitive up bows with his arm when I encourage him to play on his own without my help.

It might sound trite, but there's truth to the saying "the eyes are the window to the soul." Alex's eyes say so much about what he's thinking and wanting and trying to convey. Since that first day we met when I thought about how we'd celebrate all his progress, no matter how small that progress or no matter how it came about, I've known that having the opportunity to co-create a style of learning that works for him would stretch and inspire both of us.

After Alex clearly conveyed the motion and direction of an up and down bow, we traced the bow along the path he created in his own way. I loved that Alex discovered a way to respond with a fabulous application and demonstration of his understanding.

I have to admit that, even though I've never had any doubts about Alex's ability to learn, I have had—and still, occasionally, do have—doubts about my ability to teach a student whose learning style requires greater innovation and aptitude.

In the very early days of Alex and my working together, I called to a former undergraduate colleague of mine, looking for some creative and adaptive ideas that would help in my lessons with Alex.

"So," I began, excitedly. "I've got this great little fourth grader who wants to learn the cello, and he has Down Syndrome and—"

But before I could finish my sentence, they dismissively responded, "Well if he isn't making progress then don't feel bad about telling his parents that it's just not working out. You've already got a busy schedule with all those schools and..."

Their voice suddenly felt far away as my ears began to burn with anger and my mind raced. What made them assume Alex wasn't going to make progress? Why wouldn't I have time for this student? *I'm a string teacher, this is what I'm meant to have time for,* I thought indignantly. Did this fellow teacher think I was coming to them to...*complain*? To find a way out of teaching Alex?

I felt defensive of my new cello student, and this encounter only made me feel more determined to shatter expectations. *Alex can do this.* But that didn't mean I didn't feel personally inadequate. Would I be able to give Alex what he deserved? I was a new teacher after all, with such little experience and my special education training consisted of one short semester of Music in Special Education.

And yet, I'd come to learn that Alex and his team of supports—especially Nancy—have graciously taught me how to teach Alex.

In March 2020, the COVID-19 pandemic arrived and our in-person lessons changed to virtual lessons for over a year and a half, which made seeing the nuances in Alex's expressions and feeling the small micro-movement initiations in his hands and arms difficult for me. But Nancy's attunement to her son's movements and reactions were a tremendous asset. The three of us—Alex and Nancy at their home, and me on the other side of the screen—adapted to this now virtual world.

One way we adapted was by using a cello stand to hold Alex's cello. By using the cello stand, Nancy was able to sit to his side while guiding his arms, essentially clearing the way for more support and interaction with Alex as he engaged with his cello. Though virtual lessons had many non-ideal speedbumps along the way—like not being able to as easily follow Alex's cues, and all the glitchy delays with the sound and video—I felt I could use the virtual platform to my advantage and begin focusing more on teaching Alex about note reading.

Luckily, just before the pandemic, I had color coded each of his four open strings with a sticker on the fingerboard, just beneath the strings at eye level for Alex. To introduce him to the concept of note reading, I had begun to try to use squares and rectangles of matching color-coded construction paper.

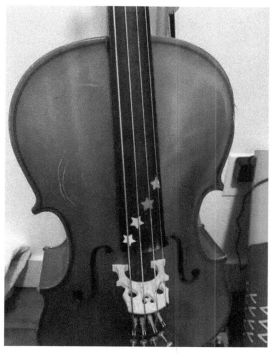

Alex's color-coded cello. I also used the positioning of the stickers to represent the lowness or highness of the string's pitch.

For example, a red square was a short red note (red is his open A string), and a blue rectangle is a long blue note (blue is his open D string), and so on with his green G string and yellow C string. I'd sing a pattern to Alex and dance the coordinated colorful shapes in the air to the beat in front of him. Nancy would sit beside him and help him follow along with his bow or *pizzicato* fingers. With this strategy, I once again felt like I needed another pair of arms as the pieces of paper would go flying from my hands, whirling around us as Alex tossed his bow to the floor. I love that Nancy has a great sense of humor. We would often find ourselves laughing at our own unique struggles during these lessons

In a way, the Zoom lessons alleviated the need for Nancy and me to become construction paper contortionists, and I instead wrote the notes out on a music staff in a more traditional fashion, yet still with color coordination. Each new song or pattern we learned got a matching, color-coded note, and I'd share my screen over Zoom, encouraging Alex to begin to track the notes as he played. Since we'd been working only with his four open strings in his learning so far, his patterns and songs usually consisted of about two to three notes that bob up or down on the staff to match the pitch he sees and hears.

Nancy has been amazing at thinking about and finding seating arrangements that will keep Alex at eye level with his points of contact on the cello (his color-coded stickers and/or his bow contact point on the strings between the bridge and fingerboard), as well as keeping him supported by making sure his feet are grounded. Nancy shared with me that this is called proximal stability, a concept I'd never heard spoken about in that way but with which I'd had experience because of my own experience as a musician.

I've always known that being physically grounded is essential when playing an instrument. Many of my teachers would remind me to keep my feet flat and secure on the earth, but Nancy gave me language for a concept I'd used without being able to describe. Alex is living it, too. Proximal stability allows for the music to flow through him, and starting with a strong root to the earth helps him support his core so that everything extending from it will have a reliable support to stem and move from.

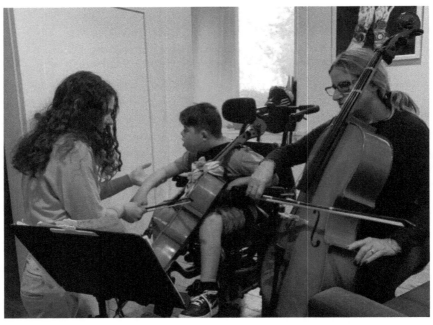

Alex using his wheelchair to support his core and feet during a cello lesson.

9 Nancy

When I received the instrument interest form, with its single question—Which instrument would you like your child to learn?—and limited multiple-choice answers, I thought He's not going to be able to do any of these things, so why are they even bothering to send this to me?

Waves of frustration washed over me. Throughout my years with Alex, I've marveled at my youngest son's abilities, joys and radiant spirit, but that doesn't mean I don't feel frustrated when he can't do the things his peers seem so easily able to accomplish. I'm never sad about my son's limitations for me, but I do want him to experience a wider, more expansive life, and reminders of what he can't do make me sad and angry. The form felt mean.

Alex didn't walk—yet. Or talk—yet. He found it challenging to hold a pencil. There was no way he'd be able to join the orchestra.

My heart sank, and then it soared. What if Alex could experience even some small measure of music? What if he could learn to play? Here was the opportunity for a new experience, and I didn't want my youngest deprived of anything.

Josh played the cello. I played, and still sometimes play, the cello. I wished Alex could play the cello. So, I pushed down my doubts. I filled in the box marked "cello."

Another form showed up the next day. It instructed me to rent a quarter-size cello.

Really? Well, here goes. I rushed to the Music and Arts store in Wayne, Pennsylvania.

"I need a quarter-size cello, a bow, some rosin, and Suzuki book one," I told the young man behind the counter.

He wrote Alex in big black letters on a tag and attached the tag to the soft instrument case. I thought about the letters we'd hung on my third son's bedroom door, even before bringing him home from the hospital, and smiled at the inner acknowledgement of how our lives with Alex had far exceeded our expectations. Alex had exceeded our expectations. But, as I left the music store, clutching Alex's instrument to me, I was far from confident.

And yet...

The pictures were sent to me of Alex taking his first lesson with his cello teacher, April Beard. How did that happen? How did I move from uncertainty to unshakeable faith? April Beard.

April is the embodiment of all I had hoped for in a teacher. Not just for Alex, but for me.

Up until the pandemic, she sent me a weekly multi-paragraph emails about pizzicato, piano plucking with a soft dynamic level, bow holding, CelloPhant™ vs. no tool, Alex's attention span, percussion, music, and more. (After the pandemic hit, I became Alex's cello helper, so there was no need for these ongoing email updates).

To get emails about our youngest son's progress filled me with a joy that cannot be put into words. Each week, after receiving April's email, it could take me a day to respond. I remained that blown away, my doubts eviscerated by awe and gratitude. Since being blessed with the gift of my youngest son, I have felt as if I've often had to fight for him to gain access to the same rights and opportunities as his fourth-grade peers. But, with the cello, Alex is just like any other fourth grader.

April perfectly balances how to challenge Alex, yet meet him where he needs support. She turned the instrument toward him so he could see and hear. As a result of her tutelage, my son, who others doubted could ever learn to play an instrument, let alone something as intricate and majestic as a cello, can play percussion, do bouncy bowing, and so many other techniques that astonish me.

April accepts the level of learning within Alex's current reach while inspiring him to expand his skill set in increments. As a result, Alex is learning. He is also cultivating a love for music. I see this experience as setting the stage for our youngest son to touch the stars. And I marvel at what a miracle he is.

As if the photos and emails were not enough, April added to Alex's visual and textual records by beginning to video her lessons with him. Each video she sent gave us all hope and joy. I remember a day, 15 weeks into Alex's lessons, when I watched him, courtesy of one of these captured moments, and had a striking realization; Alex was progressing not just as a performer but as a person.

Alex has learned a ton about notes. He has experienced stylistic variations. His cello teacher isn't simply teaching him how to play. She is helping him understand that he can do things he never imagined

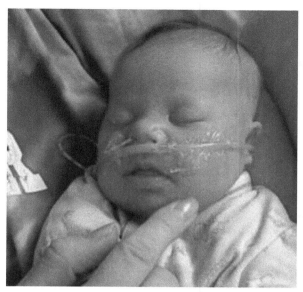

Alex was in the Bryn Mawr Hospital NICU (Newborn Intensive Care Unit) for one month after he was born.

possible. He *can* learn. This teacher's teaching has been magic. It has illuminated the intelligence we have always known Alex possesses. As a result, he is succeeding in ways I never dreamt possible, ways the world told me he never would.

At the time of Alex's birth, there were many people who told me not to have expectations for him. They said things like "I'm so sorry this happened to you," "You're going to put him in an institution, right?" and "At least, you have Josh and Sam."

They treated Alex's birth like a death and couldn't see all of the wonder and beauty that Alex would bring to our family, and, also, to the world.

Each year since then, although most of Alex's young life has been full of loving, positive people, I've found myself suddenly in situations where it feels as if other people are trying to reduce my expectations of my son. These seemingly well-intentioned people want to make Alex's life smaller. Not April. I watch, enthralled, as April issues an instruction and my youngest son takes his entire body and lifts it up higher to show he understands. An A string sounds higher than a D string.

Every time I watch Alex play, my mind wanders through a maze of memories and I find myself tearing up at the beauty and brilliance of

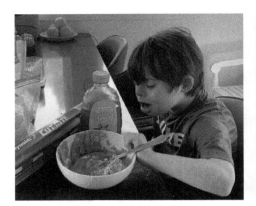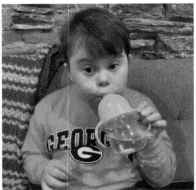

Alex helping to make Aunt Susie's peanut butter candy, and holding his own cup of water.

my youngest boy. Alex's experiences with the cello have translated into other areas of his life. Since starting the cello, his pincer grasp is better, and his grasp on life itself seems to have strengthened. He has started holding objects more at home. He looks at me with a newfound confidence and poise. It is as if, when he sees me seeing him, we both recognize that something has changed. He has an increased awareness. His sense of self and purpose have grown.

Seeing Alex respond to the notes and chords of his newfound learning fills us all with a desire to sing just as he fills our life with daily music simply by existing.

Alex:

It is so cool Miss Beard turned the cello toward me! I can see all the strings and she showed me how to get a great sound from the D string and the A string. I love this. I feel so smart and unique. I always wanted to have cello lessons. I remember Mom played the Suzuki variations of Twinkle Twinkle Little Star, and each time she played, it made me want to play too.

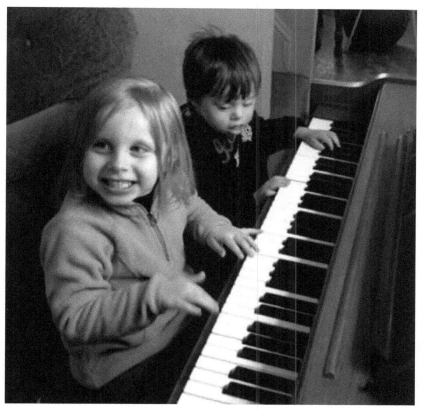

Alex playing the piano with his first friend, Fiona. They met at age four months, and are still friends at age twelve.

10 April

The practice of regularly filming Alex's lessons was a game-changer. It wasn't until six weeks into our lessons that Nancy and I thought of recording the lessons we did at school so that she could watch them at home, and I regret that I didn't get those first five lessons captured in film—although the pictures Kristen took clearly convey all of Alex's emotions. For me, teaching Alex the cello is both about how a student feels and how they develop.

I love going back and finding moments in the lesson I think are pivotal in Alex's musical development. Before Nancy began joining our in-person lessons after school just before the pandemic, and before we moved our lessons to Zoom, I would write about these developmental moments in my emails to Nancy. I used my reviews to note new opportunities for me as a teacher and to rejoice in Alex's progress. Sometimes, I find myself going back to our first recorded lessons and realizing every moment of the amazing, incremental progress Alex has made—whether it was an independent finger wiggle to initiate a pluck, or a sustained bow hold as we held a note for four beats—the video captured a lot of magic. Another beautiful result of the videos was that it allowed Nancy and her family to be able to see and share these videos. Playing music is all about sharing it with others, and, for young musicians especially, sharing music can feel like a reward.

Going to a designated music school for my undergraduate degree forced me to think of music not only as something I love, but as a calling. The responsibility to perpetuate the magnificent impact of music through the generations to come is not always talked about at the forefront of music education, but I suppose it's there at the root of every music lesson. Every up bow, every down bow. From Plato, Aristotle, and Confucius to John Adams, John F. Kennedy and Woodrow Wilson, they all understood that music education is a powerful tool in creating an intrinsically good, moral, and well-rounded society.

I think music educators can be so dedicated to their craft and students is because of how intensely we are trained to be in our often quasi conservatory-like settings. Music education degrees can be extremely rigorous and time-consuming. While musicians love music and its ability to be a means of expression, studying it, performing it, and teaching it all under deeply analytical scrutiny by your professors, peers, students and their parents, and yourself on the other side of that camcorder later on can be nearly soul-crushing at times. But then, for the love of the craft, you'd get back up in the morning, and take that band techniques class (which you spend hours upon hours a week practicing for) for a grand total of a half a credit, and then rush off to the next five half-credit courses. In music school, breakfast, lunch and dinner aren't eaten in a cafeteria or dorm room, but in a windowless practice room with a bow in one hand so you can at least practice one side of the body while the other side feeds you a sandwich. In music school, piano keys become a tempting pillow around 11:00 p.m. when that video still has to be made for Conducting 102, but maybe you can sneak in a quick nap and get it done before they kick you out of the building. In music school, friends didn't ask friends to hang out, but instead they nearly hunted you down where you've hidden somewhere between the Glazunov and Glinka scores at the music library dreading

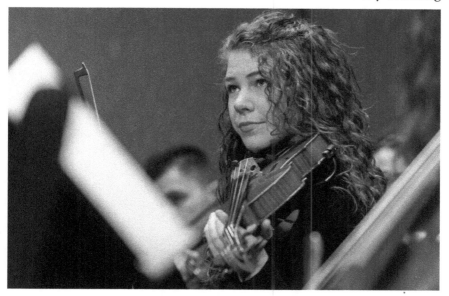

April playing viola at a rehearsal with the University of Delaware Symphony Orchestra.

that desperate ask: "Can you perform in my composition for two bassoons and a viola? When can you rehearse: after orchestra? I can do 10:00 tonight. Or what about tomorrow morning between theory and history from 8:50-9:05?" So hopeful music teachers are trained from freshman year to just go, go, go: go fill your time (constantly) with collaborating on projects, practicing, creating, teaching and hopefully, the most important thing to train in: inspiring.

Music is meant to be collaborative and every musician paves the way for those who follow.   .

After I'd been working with Alex for a while, I'd had several students with unique and individualized needs. These students all received individual lessons, but, on occasion, I would put them with other students to play. I always imagined Alex playing with his peers but, so far, his musical journey has been something different. That doesn't mean he isn't part of the orchestra community.

At Alex's elementary school during my first year, there was a moving up ceremony to celebrate the fourth graders' graduation from elementary school to middle school. I was elated when the principal asked if I could announce and acknowledge the students who participated in the orchestra. I could not wait to call the names of each of my students, watch them stand in front of their peers and parents, and see that this experience of participating in something extra, challenging, and special was important and deserved recognition after all. I read the name "Alexander Schwartz," and glancing up from the speaker's podium to watch Kristen help raise him up. He stood as the audience clapped, and I felt so proud of him. I knew that he felt proud too.

Each week, before sending Nancy the video link, I'd watch back through Alex's lesson and notice moments that I thought were important then point them out to her in an accompanying email. I owe my video analysis skills to my undergraduate professors. My viola professor, Dr. T, had me record each one of my weekly viola lessons with her, watch them back, and write a reflection paper on my observations and insights. Though sometimes tedious, the information gained from this exercise was powerful. In a similar fashion, in our community string teaching practicum called the National String Project Consortium, every lesson I taught was recorded, watched back, and reflected upon in written form.

Being able to watch myself teaching and analyze how my approach did or didn't impact a student was humbling and informative. I could see what worked and what really engaged each particular student. Equally valuable was seeing what didn't.

Sometimes watching back lessons reveals missed opportunities. It only takes a few times seeing a missed opportunity before you realize the sacredness of your role as a teacher and how essential it is to run with the magic your students are giving you. I think one of my favorite parts of teaching is when I let students inspire their lessons. I never mind "de-railing" from the lesson plan because a student asks an "unrelated" question. After all, to me, and what I'd love to teach all my students, is that music is related to everything, and everything can be related to music.

I've been in the midst of demonstrating a basic string playing technique and had plenty of students suddenly ask how to play "Happy Birthday" for their mom this weekend, or "What is that cool finger wiggle thing you do sometimes?", and what follows is pure perfection. Every curiosity or question provides an opportunity to learn. In fact, the more free a student feels to ask about seemingly "unrelated" questions, the more they can translate what they're learning from their engagement with music into the rest of their life.

Sometimes, I marvel at my cat, Marty. When he falls from a surface, he is able to turn mid-air within a matter of milliseconds before hitting the ground so he can land safely on his feet. To me, this has become a metaphor for teaching music. Sometimes, when I'm working with Alex, the lesson plan falls through for a moment because Alex's expression, posture, or reaction to a cue pushes us in a new direction. With a little creativity, love and passion for the subject, we can pivot and connect Alex's student-sprung inspiration to a meaningful moment of learning. I've found that the more easily I learn to pivot along with a student, the less friction and frustration. I almost never get frustrated with my students—they're all such wonderful sponges for learning—but I have to confess that I do occasionally get frustrated with myself when I'm having a hard time nudging them out of a plateau or helping them meet that next stage of their musical development.

One of the things I've really appreciated about working with Alex has been that I had no expectations, and the agenda is always pushing forward, or there's no shame in falling back to review some skill when needed.

The beginning lessons with Alex were exploratory. My only goals were to inspire him to think, *Hmmm…what kind of noise can I make with this thing? When I do this, it sounds like that…so what happens if*

I do this? and to allow him to experiment with the unfamiliar in an environment that fostered exploration and curiosity.

Independent movement and action initiated by Alex quickly became, and have remained, big goals for him, not simply in music but in all areas of his life. Letting Alex initiate movement and interaction with the cello is important. In our early days together, I would guide his hand towards the cello and let his thumb rest on the string until he was ready to tug at it and pluck. As I learned to read the music of Alex's expressions and initiations, I noticed that sometimes he initiates with his left hand and sometimes with his right. He is an ambidextrous explorer of his instrument and his surroundings. Once again, Alex's unique needs and learning style set our course rather than what I thought we were "supposed" to do.

When we first began our lessons, I decided I had to let go of the "rule" that Alex should only pluck and bow with his right hand, even though I firmly hold on to this rule for all my other students. Because of the way the instruments are built from the inside out, the violin, viola, cello and double bass are made to play with the left hand holding the instrument and the right hand plucking or bowing. It's possible to play the other way around I suppose, but you'd typically only ever see people playing in an alternative way if they have a significant reason for doing so, such as following a stroke, or a limb amputation.

I have students who protest that they are left or right-handed and that means they should hold their instrument opposite of what I'm instructing, but the funny thing is, it doesn't really matter if you are dominant with your left or right hand; either way, you need both hands to play! Both hands perform equally important duties simultaneously and they rely on each other to make music. Both hands are rhythmic, expressive, and dictate pretty much everything in the music in conjuncttion with each other.

But Alex's journey with the cello is (in regards to posture, not in regards to all things) is different from all my other students. When I first started Alex on the cello, essentially, *I* was holding the cello in a traditional setup, while Alex engaged with the cello from the front. His major goals during his first formative lessons were to:

- Observe how the cello makes sound and in what ways he can control the sound

- Visually and aurally identify and sustain contact with the four strings

- Work on the fine-motor coordination needed for plucking the strings

- Track the bow directions (up bow and down bow)

- Maintain a bow hold with assistance, and eventually without

At the very beginning, I was less flexible about which hand Alex used to do what. I was initially pretty insistent about him only using the right hand for plucking and bowing as he would if he were holding the cello the traditional way. When I'd felt like it was a challenge for Alex to sustain actions for more than a few moments with his right hand, I had asked Kristen which hand Alex used most often. She told me he tends to favor the left hand, so I guess it was out of curiosity and some realization that there'd be a need for flexibility in Alex's lessons, that I followed Alex's initiation and lead as he reached out with his left hand to grab the strings during one lesson. Alex initiating and engaging became a more important skill to me than putting up the barriers of which hand does which. So, from there on, he seemed to initiate with the left hand often, but sometimes also with the right hand. Or sometimes his left hand would get tired midway through the lesson so we'd switch over to the right hand pretty seamlessly.

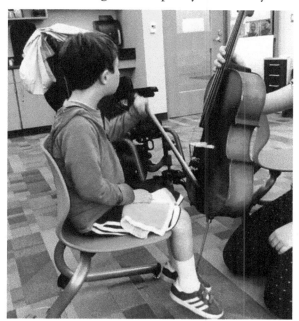

Alex during one of his 4th grade lessons, holding the bow in his left hand while the cello faced him.

While I teach a lot of the same concepts to Alex as I do my other students, Nancy, Alex and I envision his experience with the cello to be a physical, spiritual, mental discovery of movement, exercise, and the creation of an expressive art. For Alex, perhaps more so than for many of my other students, music is a vehicle for learning so many other life skills that use motor coordination. Learning skills that use movement in his hands and arms is a large focus. It took a few lessons for me to change my thinking, but it wasn't long before I decided to switch from "let's not use that hand because that's the wrong one" to "Oh, you'd like to use this hand now? Okay, why not! Let's apply the same skills from the left to the right now."

I often say that I learn more from Alex than he learns from me. Some of the biggest lessons so far are to let go of my inflexibility and self-consciousness. And the left/right hand switching, while against the "rules," wasn't against the intention of increased agility and physical balance, which all musicians are encouraged to cultivate. When Alex began switching hands, I thought of the Alexander Technique. "The Alexander Technique is an educational method used worldwide for well over 100 years. By teaching how to change faulty postural habits, it enables improved mobility, posture, performance, and alertness along with relief of chronic stiffness, tension, and stress" (American Society for the Alexander Technique™).

Developing some ambidextrousness is a concept I was already familiar with through the Alexander Technique. If we can consciously begin integrating our non-dominant side into everyday life, it helps to help create greater balance and ease of movement.

Trying daily tasks with your non-dominant side of the body—like opening a door or brushing your hair—is a practice I occasionally think about from my Alexander studies. The thought is that doing so can bring more body awareness, and you can observe your level of balance and harmony between the two sides. There is no vertical line dividing the body in half. It's one body that needs to work in harmony.

In cello playing, the left and right sides are used in completely different ways, but they are both being used with equal importance.

I asked myself, "Is Alex still working toward and making progress with his goals no matter the hand?" And the answer: Yes! And that eased some of that worry that I was teaching him "all wrong." Yet...

One day while we were still doing virtual lessons, Nancy asked me if I thought Alex was ready to turn the cello around to be more like the traditional set up. He was becoming stronger, more confident, and though I didn't know if there'd ever be that clear moment where I'd think he's ready, I envisioned Alex sitting with his cello, the fingerboard swung over his left shoulder as traditional, while the right hand plucks and bows...

Relief. I felt relief just thinking about Alex holding that cello like every other cellist. That is definitely the classically trained musician in me, along with fear of being a "bad teacher" or seeming unknowledgeable about the performance of string instruments. However, beyond those sort of selfish reasons, educationally for Alex, I did begin to think that finally turning things around would be a great springboard for future skills like using the left hand to plop down on the strings to make new notes. It would also allow him to rest his arm and hand weight into the strings, using gravity to play in a relaxed and naturally supported way. I would imagine it would also strengthen Alex's observational connection from what he sees when Nancy or me show him videos of other cellists playing.

I often tell my students that playing a string instrument is like patting your head with one hand and rubbing your belly with the other at the same time... while also spinning plates on your nose, hopping on one foot, and reciting the alphabet backward. There's a lot going on, which makes learning, practicing, and playing an instrument physically and mentally stimulating and healthy, as well as an intricate balancing act. In Alex's case, learning to play the cello has become its own kind of physical therapy and has helped strengthen his muscles and coordination skills. Playing a string instrument can do this for everyone, and the reason why the body and string instruments are so linked is because the more aligned and relaxed your body is, the more beautiful your sound will be. Music falls into alignment when you are aligned. If your body is in a reliable position, you can be more rhythmic and reliable with your intonation, inflection, and shifts from note to note, and from position to position. Reliable positions are tension-free and as neutral as possible. This is much easier said than done, because of all that head patting, belly rubbing, plate spinning, hopping, reading, interpreting, decoding, deciding, and expressing that you're expected to be doing...and sometimes while in front of an audience. But that's where practicing correct form is essential.

My teachers always reminded me about my feet first, which is why I always appreciate Nancy's efforts to make sure Alex has proximal stability by giving his feet contact to the ground or to a stable surface. From there, we can align his body all the way upwards through his

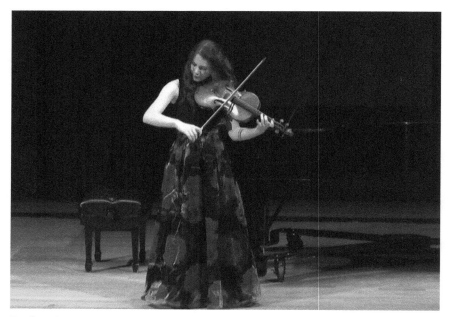

Performing with body awareness and alignment so that the music flows as naturally as possible

springy knees, curvy spine, and open-hearted torso. Achieving proximal stability is different for every musician, and even different for the same musician, depending on the day.

Because the Alexander Technique was available to me through both degrees (both of my college music programs had an accessible Alexander teacher, probably non-coincidentally), I've been educated in environments that emphasize the relationship between music and physicality. Then again, Frederick Matthias Alexander, creator of the Alexander Technique, was himself a vocalist so he always saw a connection between music, the body, and performance. Along with addressing techniques to improve body awareness, the Alexander Technique can address performance anxiety as well. In fact, my increased ability to rely on my body awareness and alignment helped with my ability to be calm on stage during solo recitals. From the shy girl I once was, to someone who's learned to perform over hour-long recitals solo on stage, I've been able to use physical grounding techniques to give myself permission to relax under pressure, and in public.

Because there is so much going on when playing an asymmetrical string instrument, we tend to tense up in areas where there is really no need to tense up in, and we experience pain either while playing or after playing. Unfortunately, we've all had scenarios and activities in our lives that have caused us to develop this tension, whether it be from an accident or an injury, or from simply performing a mundane task like typing, or texting on a phone. Not only did the Alexander Technique help me realize in what areas I could release tension, but my teachers could also identify places where I would be squeezing or clenching through my playing either visually, kinesthetically, or even audibly. In fact, when a musician is struggling to make progress in a skill or technique, it will often be because of tension.

For Alex, whose Trisomy 21 is correlated with hypotonia, there is no denying the correlation between musculature and music. His hypotonia means the two of us, aided by Nancy, need to understand and gauge his levels of strength and flexibility within his arms, hands, and shoulders at each and every lesson. For this reason, and other reasons like instilling a sense of independence and initiation, Nancy and I never want to force Alex to do a movement on the cello when we guide him. Like in my own viola playing and to all my students, I try to refer to actions on the strings as "weighing down" or "weight." Our arms, hands and the bow obviously all have weight to them, so using the natural weight of the bow and arm into the string is helpful for both those who tend to tense up, and for those who perhaps have a condition like Alex where the muscles may not always be able to consistently activate. For the most part, we are able to rest. And though that is another surprisingly "easier said than done" thing, resting the arm and bow, and letting gravity do the work, is an important skill to learn.

Watching old lessons with Alex enabled me to pick up on subtle cues and shifts not merely in his movements, but in his pre-movements. I think it's kind of like how when anyone's listening to music, most people can almost subconsciously predict when a chord is about to change, or when the chorus is about to come back in, or when the beat will "drop." We feel the buildup of music, and I could see Alex becoming ready for movements in tandem with the repetitive movements we practiced, or an auditory cue. The additional gift of the videos was that, in sharing the videos with Nancy, it began to feel like we were, and are, two maestros conducting a beautiful symphony together, noticing and pointing out all of Alex's cool learning moments.

After Nancy watched each lesson, she provided information that has helped me learn more about Alex and the ways he communicates. For example, she shared with me how blowing raspberries means he's

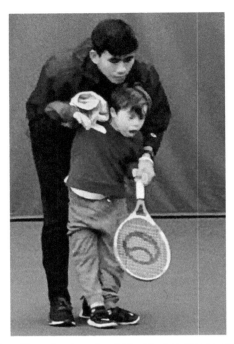

Dylan helps Alex play tennis at the Radnor Racquet Club.

loving what he's doing, and tapping his chin with his fingers in the shape of the letter "W" means he's thirsty. She pointed out that he raises his body up when he hears a higher pitch. She'd take screenshots from the videos and say, "Look how proud he looks!" Through her eyes, I started to see and learn how expressive Alex is. Ultimately, that unlocked a whole vault of knowledge and "assessment tools," where I could watch Alex and assess his ways of applying knowledge and showing understanding. I began to realize the various ways Alex is conducting and co-creating, like a third conductor in our symphony, and I became more adept at taking my cues from him.

Nancy would share with me other experiences Alex was having outside of his lessons—like swimming, basketball, or tennis. Once I knew Alex was participating in these experiences with his family each week, I could incorporate that language into his weekly cello lesson. Nancy would share music that she played for Alex that week, and we could build off that in our lessons. One week, he listened to a Bach cello suite in the car and at home, so we played open strings along to the Bach Cello Suite at his lesson. Later on in our Zoom lessons, I developed a color coded "Bach Pattern" that mimicked the slurred bow movement and string crossing coordination of the famous *Prélude* of the first Bach Cello Suite. Practicing this pattern was a great way for Alex to work on things like wrist and elbow flexibility. As I described the pattern and rationale for practicing it to Nancy over Zoom one day, I realized just how this partnership, friendship, and mentorship relationship with Nancy was—and is—pivotal in Alex's musical development. And to me too. The year I began teaching Alex was my first year teaching full-time in a public school setting and, although I felt abuzz with possibility, I didn't really know whether or not I'd be able to give my students the same level of instruction that they might have received from a more seasoned teaching veteran. But thankfully, Nancy's encouragement and support were ubiquitous from our very first lesson.

I've said before that Alex was a gift to my school district's orchestra program, and I think it's important to articulate how and why, specifically, Alex became a role model for his peers. With every up bow and down bow, he was saying to his fellow students "Look! You can do anything!"

As Alex soared, he showed others that they could do the same—including me. I still don't have the specific qualifications or certifications that would say to the world *I'm equipped to teach students with special needs*, but I now have important experience that has given me a small, yet essential, measure of self-trust.

After I'd been working with Alex for a while, I gained students who needed various accommodations for learning their instruments due to challenges such as Cerebral Palsy, Autism Spectrum Disorder, and fine-motor coordination delays. Many students have IEPs (Individualized Education Programs) and some have 504 Education Plans (plans that protect students by allowing for accommodations in any classroom environment, even at the collegiate level). All of my students are brilliant and beautifully talented members of my little beginner orchestras. I'm not sure if some of them, or some of their parents, would have signed up to work with me had Alex not paved the way as a pioneer to innovation and individual exploration.

One day, Nancy sent me a text message about Gustavo Dudamel, an enormous advocate of music education for the children of Venezuela and a brilliant, world-renowned conductor. I have always admired him for the work he's done to make music education—and specifically learning and playing a string instrument—accessible to underprivileged communities. She said she loved his philosophy of giving every child access to beauty and how *all* children deserve and have a right to beautiful experiences.

Every morning, at each school, I stand in the hallways to greet students as they come in the building. I look at each child as a potential future musician, no matter what their circumstances.

Alex has shown me, has shown his family, and has shown his entire school community that yes, each and every one of them *can* do it. They can squeeze every last bit of knowledge and skill out of learning an instrument and grow beyond whatever arbitrary musical barriers others have imposed on them. That's what Alex has done, and will continue to do. One of my favorite children's books is *If You Give a Mouse a Cookie* by Laura Numeroff. I think: if you give a child an instrument, they'll ask you to learn music. And if you give them some music, they'll give so much beauty back to you, and to the world, and what is more magical than that?

11   **Nancy**

On Alex's first day of cello lessons, his amazing personal care assistant and our lifelong family friend, Kristen Culligan, captured his elated joy in photographs. She was just as excited as our whole family for Alex to begin his cello lessons, and, after Kristen sent the photos to Kim Gambone, Alex's special education teacher, Kim forwarded the photographs to me. I cried. I cry at everything, so that wasn't new. What was new was seeing Alex light up, his smile stretching across his face, his body almost bouncy with exuberance. My youngest son does not smile and laugh easily. To evoke that level of joy, it has to be a banana, a milkshake, or the cello. And, because Alex's smiles are so rare, they're almost like watching the sunrise. I mean, sure, the sun comes up daily, but even though I wake up around 4 am each day, I'm rarely ever outside to see it.

In advance of Alex's first lesson, Kim Gambone made sure to reach out to April so that April felt supported.

> Hi April,
>
> I'm Alex's multiple disabilities teacher, Kim Gambone, I'm so excited for Alex to take cello lessons with you! I was looking at his schedule and I think 3:10 pm to dismissal would be great on Mondays as you suggested. If that time still works for you, let me know. Also, Alex will have an aide with him during the lesson. She knows him very well, so if you have any questions about his learning styles, etc… she is a great resource. Feel free to also touch base with me about anything you need.

When I was attending Teachers College at Columbia University, my professor, Cornelius Minor, told us, "The quality of relationships in a school is directly proportional to the quality of the education happening there." Alex has been fortunate to be surrounded by people who have embraced not only information, but the unique needs and learning styles of each child they educate. When facing a daunting challenge, it is essential to have support. I've been lucky to have found a lot of support, both for myself as a person and in my role as a parent. It's not always in the moment that I realize how invaluable every person's contribution is, or every incremental improvement. For example, when I watched Alex's early lessons, I wouldn't have always seen Alex's improvements, if April hadn't pointed them out to me. I saw my son happy and eager—and that felt like enough—but it's only been through time, and hindsight, that I've come to appreciate the scope of Alex's musical transformation. It reminds me of my middle son, Sam.

Because his brother, Josh, had already achieved physical benchmarks before him, Sam felt an inner drive to walk, run, and play so he could join in his older brother's fun. I can recall times when it was as if he was preparing himself to become capable of something—like walking—before he actually did it. It took him actually walking for me to realize, *He's been envisioning and striving for this all along.*

There's a young man with Down syndrome, Chris Nikic, who completed the Ironman in 2020. At 21 years of age, he made history as the first person with Down syndrome to complete an Ironman triathlon.

Guinness World Records recognized Nikic's achievement after he finished a 2.4-mile swim, a 112-mile bike ride and a 26.2-mile marathon run at the Ironman Florida competition in Panama City Beach, and the story appeared throughout local and national news outlets. Most people would not attempt an Ironman, let alone complete it and, in a podcast interview, Chris' dad said that what it took was the ability to get "1% better each day."

Chris' story makes each cell in my body feel that anything is possible, and, like Chris' dad, I believe we each get better each day. But I would also add that we can't get better alone. We need a team to wrap around ourselves like a warm blanket on a cold day.

April's response to Kim's was equally kind and supportive:

> Fabulous! Let's plan on Mondays at 3:10 pm. I have plenty of rosin. I will be looking at getting him some adaptive tools to help make the cello more comfortable.

Alex is now in his third year of studying the cello with April. Working collaboratively, we have found lots of adaptive tools. A cello stand helped support the cello upright for Alex when we transitioned to virtual lessons.

That doesn't mean Alex isn't still receiving external support. It just looks a little different. For instance, I invited his occupational therapist, Kasey, to sit in on Zoom lessons to get her feedback. At a recent lesson, she suggested applying pressure to his finger as he plucks (*pizzicato*) on the string to give his finger input, which has helped create a richer sound. Soon, Alex's physical therapist will watch a lesson to see how we can create less distance between him and his cello.

While the pandemic has been horrible, one small, beautiful miracle to come to us during this time has been that I've gotten to be at Alex's side for all of his cello lessons and observe his progress in a different, more hands-on way.

With each passing week, it seems we are constantly evaluating ergonomics, positionality, and proximal stability. We meet one challenge and there's another waiting. But, always, we are showered in rewards. Through a shared love of music, unending kindness, and a team approach, I am watching my youngest son blossom and grow, always in the direction of the sun.

Alex:

GaGa (my word for my grandma) gets happy when mom shows her my cello lessons in the video Ms. Beard sends. I feel proud that GaGa is watching me play. I know she knows I can do it too. My other grandma, Grandma JoAnne, cried when she saw it, I think it made her happy too. I wish I could keep my grasp on my bow longer.

12 April

In February of 2021, we began having Alex sit with the cello with the traditional set up while he is supported in his wheelchair. After two years of having the instrument face him, the back of the cello now rests on his sternum, with his knees gently positioned on either side of the cello. We strive to maintain an angle that allows the neck of the cello to swing over his left shoulder, because this positioning allows his left hand to maneuver more naturally. This has required some trial and error with the positioning of the instrument, Alex's body, and his wheelchair.

Alex sits in his wheelchair with a brace to help him sit up as the cello leans into him. The best part for me as Alex's teacher was to discover that the transition to this "new" set up was not as gradual or shocking as I had thought it would be for Alex. In fact, he's taken much of what he's learned with the cello strings facing him and applied it to the strings facing outward. I was inspired to make this transition after a conversation with Nancy.

"I think he's ready," she told me when I asked for her opinion. "He's stronger and he's got way better arm extension."

She was right. Nowadays, Alex's arms are stronger and more mobile in extended positions, and he is navigating around to the strings—with some help from Nancy—quite beautifully, and with less support. He's working on supporting the cello at the bout (the place where the neck meets the body, almost like the shoulders of the cello) with his left hand, which he is wonderfully sustaining for most of the lesson, and we are bowing with his right hand. We use his thumb and pointer fingers in varying plucking patterns. He works on strumming across the strings with his thumb, and when plucking strings individually, he works on anchoring the thumb to the fingerboard while the pointer finger reaches across to tug at each string.

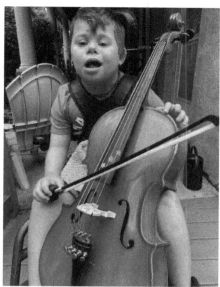

Alex now sitting with the cello in the traditional posture.

I think posture and setup are an ongoing journey for all string players. Our bodies change, even day to day; somedays we are tired—our shoulders feel heavy, or we slept at a strange angle—and somedays we feel anxious or energetic and we compensate with tight muscles and stiff limbs. Each day, each lesson, Alex adjusts to find the most natural positioning possible for his body at the present moment. When we were in-person and he'd come for his lesson, Kristen would update me on how his day had been and, at home, over Zoom with Nancy, she offers a quick Alex's day update each time we commence a lesson. For all students, it's essential to be attuned to their current physical state but it's especially so for those who require physical assistance. Because we only ever want to support Alex's movements, we need to be attuned to his needs, which change based on innumerable variables.

In this next picture, we captured Alex beginning to initiate a fabulous hold on the neck and fingerboard. What's especially notable about this is how he immediately began forming a natural "cup holding" shape with his thumb about opposite his middle two fingers. Beyond that, we will begin expanding his knowledge and skills to include tapping on the strings, and eventually plopping his fingers down on the strings to create more notes. But, as it is, there is no shortage of things to try and ways to grow. We've begun to regularly incorporate an exercise in which Nancy uses her own pointer finger to act like a

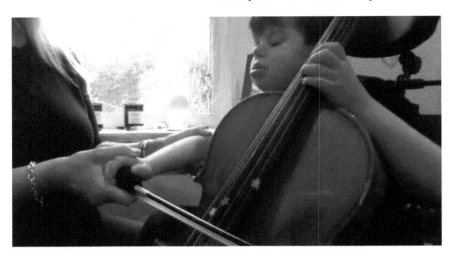

Nancy helping Alex sustain a grasp on the bow, while he works on left hand positioning on the fingerboard.

lever under Alex's fingers and help him feel the motion of lifting and dropping fingers from his left hand base knuckles.

Alex has often made me think about how lucky those of us are who find instruments and are able to play music as a way to work on ourselves. Music is no doubt a kind of physical therapy, but with my one semester of Music in Special Education, and no background or degree in music therapy, I can only hope that what I lack in experience I make up for in enthusiasm.

I still often feel a sense of "imposter syndrome." I know that someone out there is more qualified, more knowledgeable, more *actually* certified to teach Alex music than I am, and I often feel very, very undeserving of the praise Nancy gives me. I know I'm missing a whole catalogue of knowledge, vocabulary, and strategies that a music therapist would know like the back of their hand. What I do have, however, are the two most important words I learned during that one semester of Music in Special Education: *adaptions* and *accommodations*. I do my best to adapt and accommodate in order to give Alex a meaningful, musical experience.

Whenever I focus on my own limitations as a teacher, which I do more than I care to admit, I try to remember that I am doing my best and that, just as I am proud of Alex, I want to strive to appreciate my own accomplishments in the face of what others might view as my limitations. I have to say that I'm not as good at celebrating myself as I am at celebrating Alex. But what has been different for me, and what

I've been able to not only accept but embrace, has been this new-found team approach to teaching.

When we were doing virtual lessons, Nancy invited Alex's teachers, occupational therapist, and physical therapist to periodically join and be a part of our lessons, and the knowledge and experience I gained from them is invaluable. Nancy is an incredibly loving, knowledgeable and caring mother, and her communication, support, and engagement in this process have been indispensable, both to me and to Alex. I am an expert in music, yes, but she is an expert in her son, and it is through her and the other members of Alex's "village" and Alex's upbeat attitude, teachability and persistence, that he is achieving and exceeding every goal. Alex is bringing music to life.

It helps that Nancy is an educator herself. But I think it's part of her personality to make those around her feel valued and loved. This was immediately clear upon first meeting her in person, when she enveloped me in a huge hug, thanked me for bringing music into Alex's life, then launched into a rush of conversation as though we were old friends. By that point in time we were old friends, even if we'd only ever communicated via email. Nancy is an avid emailer, which has been hugely helpful considering that parental support and communication have been key factors in the success of Alex's lessons. Nancy and her love of Alex and the cello has been Alex's biggest ally as he's embarked on what some said was impossible.

Alex is a musician with unlimited potential. Beyond that, he is a student who inspires me, and beyond even that, he is a student who gives me a greater sense of purpose by bringing to life a teaching philosophy I believe in more and more with each passing day. Nancy has also continuously inspired me and given me a greater sense of purpose as an educator. As an educator herself, as well as a mother, she demonstrates by example a willingness to adapt her approach to inspire those around her to learn and grow. She is constantly challenging herself to create opportunities for growth and self-expression.

I want to continue to learn and grow as a teacher, make connections and form relationships with as many brilliant people as I can, sharing and gaining ideas and knowledge along the way. I want to do for others what Alex and his circle of supports, especially his mother, have done for me.

13 Nancy

Years ago, I was fortunate to be able to see Carol Ann Tomlinson, an American educator, author and speaker, at a teacher in-service. We were all there to learn how to be better teachers, and it felt like a wonderful and rare opportunity to be in the presence of a master educator.

In order to explain the importance of differentiation, Carol invited us to think about the example of a student learning about a cell. She explained that, if a student were learning about cells and cellular structure, there would be a multitude of ways to teach and a multitude of ways for that student to show their understanding of the subject. They could write definitions, make pen and ink drawings, create a diorama, act out the reactions and interactions of the various parts of a cell, or any other number of alternatives. She urged us to remember that there are countless ways to teach and learn content, then inspired us to realize that in order to access those ways, we must broaden our reach and "think outside the box." Innovation is what keeps our world spinning. It is a gift that April is willing to not have only one way for her students to learn but a myriad of different alternatives. Together, we have come to treat Alex's cello lessons like a perpetual experiment. She is the scientist and I am her helper. Like all good scientific experiments, the most significant results are not what happens in a lab. They're what happen after the testing is over. They're what happen when you implement the skills, or the substances created, in life.

Even before we moved to Zoom and I could witness, firsthand, the magic of April's teaching, I could see the effect cello lessons were having on my third son. Since Alex cannot speak yet, he will often cry out in protest when he doesn't like something, when he's frustrated, or when he's overtired. Typically, at the end of the day, he is exhausted from his low muscle tone, and many therapies. And, usually, a class or therapy at the end of a school day would result in a loud crying episode where he would thrust both thumbs in his mouth screaming until whatever unwelcome lesson or therapy stopped. Alex has always been quite gifted at letting us know when he protests. But he's never once had a meltdown with April.

Each video of the cello lesson that April sent home, and each picture captured by Kristen, or occasionally Kim, shows a happy, compliant Alex. It is a miracle, considering that these lessons are all at the end of his school day!

Curious about Alex's positive reaction to the cello, and the joy he'd continue to display on his cello lesson days, smiling and laughing well into the evening, and grooving out to WXPN's Funky Friday playlist if I happened to put music on, I asked April how she was able to inspire my youngest son to feel excited at the end of a long, exhausting day.

"How do you get him to relax at the end of the school day? He's always so happy in the morning, but, by three, he tends to fade—fast."

April explained that music is therapy. "I'm not doing anything," she said. "Alex is doing it. He's letting the music flow through him and I'm not surprised it's having an impact."

She may not be right about her not having an impact, but April is right about Alex letting music flow through him. I see the positive impact of Alex's cello lessons as coming from love wrapped together with giving Alex a voice he did not have before. The cello lessons with April are spiritual. They allow my son to access an inner resource and to express himself in ways that he would not otherwise have access to. And Alex's capacity to relate through music, something he acquired almost immediately into their work together, has continued to expand and has permeated far beyond a single weekly 20 to 30 minute lesson.

Although April doesn't assign Alex the same set of practice exercises as to his classmates, she's encouraged our family to prioritize playing and listening to music whenever possible. We already listened a lot, but now we listen with intention.

"It's Funky Friday, Alex" or "How about some Yo-Yo Ma, Alex?" or "Are you in the mood for hip hop or classical?"

Alex loves to dance and he loves to share music with all of us. He and his brothers will listen to songs, the lyrics of which I can barely decipher, while sprawling out in Alex's bed, staring up at the ceiling or bobbing to the beat in his bedroom—which, thanks to GaGa, we were able to modify in accordance with his needs.

Michael and Alex will share alternative and retro-80s/punk-rock music whenever they're alone together and, as for me and Alex, we stick to funk and classical.

Even when our lessons were virtual, watching Alex's progress as I assist him makes me feel deep hope and joy. The lessons are magnificent. My son is magnificent.

Alex:

I looked really hard and focused on the strings Miss Beard showed me today. She was explaining how to pluck the strings, and move my bow in different directions. This is SO much fun! Sometimes I wish I could hold the cello without any help. She also explained this fancy word today. Pizzicato. It's a movement where I pluck the string and it makes this neat sound. She played Johnny Leary's Polka. It is the best. I made sure to move my thumb exactly the way Miss Beard had instructed me.

14 April

When we first started Alex's cello lessons, we used any regular class-room chairs we could find, and sometimes I even kept him in his wheelchair when we were short on time. It's funny that I used to think the wheelchair would be too restrictive, preventing Alex from being able to freely move and extend toward and around the cello. However, nowadays, after experimenting with several different chairs and confirmed by a recommendation from Alex's OT and PT support team, Nancy will move Alex to his wheelchair for our cello lessons. The support the chair gives him is so helpful, and actually frees Alex from having to worry about holding himself up while focusing on the challenging cello tasks before him.

While Alex always tried his best no matter the setup, I noticed a major improvement in his performance when we made sure his feet were planted. Yes, proximal stability is a concept with which we were familiar long before Nancy gave us the language to describe it.

For some time, we used a big, green dinosaur-inspired chair with large arm rests. The armrests worked nicely to support under his arms, but sometimes Alex would slip downward on the chair (it was more of a lounging style armchair made for children), and this would lead to him losing his eye-level connection to the strings and, therefore, losing his focus.

For any musician, no matter the instrument, setup and posture are important, and not being able to get Alex positioned optimally meant setting him up for failure rather than success. Personally, I've been so conditioned to focus on groundedness that it feels off-balanced and unfamiliar for me not to be firmly rooted prior to playing.

Every time I step foot on a stage to perform on viola, I have my teachers' voices in my head, nagging me about my feet...

"They are your root to the ground," one past teacher's voice floats by.

"They balance you all the way through your core," another says.

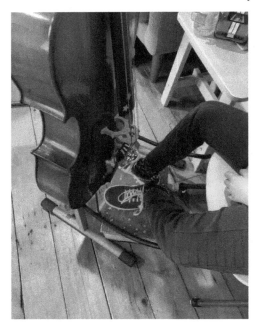
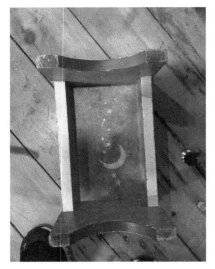

Alex using a foot bench that was hand-painted by the artist, photographer, and art educator Michelle Hollis Marsden. The bench depicts eternity in the night sky with stars from past years and a moon that shines with limitless possibility. A sun is painted on each side to remind the owner of the power of sunshine.

My feet have supported me through the asymmetry that comes with playing a string instrument. They have allowed me to plant myself where I am, but that doesn't mean it's always easy to find that sense of homeostasis. When you try to move your arms or hands in two totally different ways with varying amounts of speed, pressure, and articulation, the human body will let you know how much it does not like asymmetry. There really is very little symmetry when it comes to playing a string instrument. However, I like to think about my brief Alexander Technique learning in my schooling as a way of tapping into the versatility and dexterity of the body.

One Alexander Technique concept is to accept that most things in nature are indeed asymmetrical, and, in recognizing what our body does and is capable of, we should not be after symmetry when adjusting our posture or movements, but rather *harmony* (could there be a more perfect word?). With mindfulness, exploration, observation, and a little bit of play, we have the ability to balance ourselves in harmony so that we can move naturally, efficiently, fluidly and comfortably. When we can acknowledge that and mindfully "work" on that with our physical bodies, it is then that music can flow through us efficiently, fluidly, and naturally. That is why it is so important to spend time exploring Alex's setup with his instrument. How can we adjust his physical space to allow him to be a vehicle for his music?

When I told Nancy why Alex's movements mattered and how, from my standpoint, proximal stability was simply one component of a larger drive toward body harmony, she was not only fascinated by, but familiar with, the concept. She told me that, as a little girl, she'd learned the Alexander Technique from an expert to help alleviate her neck pain. Then she said something that I hadn't thought of, but which seemed symbolically significant:

"How amazing that a technique named with my son's name would later help him in his pursuit of learning the cello!"

15   **Nancy**

I have always been a gifted communicator. Whether by phone, text, email, "snail" mail, or face-to-face conversation, I want to share my thoughts and have others share with me. Communication is everything. It keeps us all connected. Being seen and being heard are essential for all of us. Because Alex does not speak yet, I am his voice. Michael is his voice. His brothers, Josh and Sam, are his voice. The cello gives Alex a voice.

Sam is the president of his national honor society at his high school and is getting ready to give a speech. When I asked him what he would share in his speech he said, "I'm going to talk about unity. Unity is the state of being united or joined. We are all in this world of ours connected through communication."

One of many things I've learned from Alex is that his nonverbal communication can say as much—or sometimes even more—as I can say with my words. We all have our own unique ways of expressing ourselves and understanding others. Even before the Tobii and its eye-gaze technology, Alex spoke to me in non-verbal ways, ways that required a deeper level of listening. Something that was a challenge for me when Alex first went to school, and began to be taken care of by those outside our immediate family, was wondering *Will people understand him? Will they have the skills to hear him and meet his needs?*

The irony is that Alex's circle of supporters has helped me to better understand my son, to discern his messages, and to express his experiences. I've learned more about Alex by seeing him reflected through the eyes of others who love him.

One of my favorite ways to hear about my son is through emails from Alex's teachers—all his many teachers and those spearheading his various therapies—or through the brief (pre-COVID) early-morning or end-of-day drop-off, or pick-up debriefings.

Being with Alex every day, I can sometimes miss out on his incremental changes, but these trained practitioners don't. They see what I can't, and they also reaffirm what I'm noticing on my own. Of all the communications and interactions, April's emails, and now our shared Zoom time with Alex, tend to be my favorite. The emails are especially precious. I return to them sometimes after Alex has one of his nocturnal seizures, or when he's hitting a wall in another area of his life. Not only do April's emails contain hope, but they demonstrate her respect for Alex as a cello student. Regardless of his abilities, she sees his gifts.

Whenever I opened one of April's emails, they struck me as the typical emails any mom of a fourth-grade student would receive from her child's cello teacher. This type of "regular" is as rare as a shooting star. To me, a mom who often receives emails containing IEPs as thick as the Otzarreta Forest in Spain notes outlining the need for new MAFO's (Molded Ankle-Foot Orthosis, which are braces to keep Alex's knees from getting injured due to his severe hypotonia) costing $1,200, messages about wheelchair adjustment appointments that last longer than a movie table reading, doctor's messages, medication changes, confirmations for ARC provider meetings that never stop and have yet to provide meaningful support, waiver signups, and so many more reminders of challenges, stressors, and logistical nightmares, I cherished April's emails. Much like the style she uses to teach Alex the cello, April's emails became light sparkling in hope to my soul. There was magic in them.

Hi there! So glad Alex could make it back in time for his lesson today!

I just wanted to let you know that today we found it might be best if Alex tried playing the cello with the strings facing him. We only tried this with plucking, but he focuses his attention more on the strings and is able to use his left hand to pluck if we spin it around this way. We can see how this plays out with the bow next week!

Thank you and have a great evening,

April

Hi Mrs. Schwartz,

Today's cello lesson went very well! I think having the cello turned toward him is working great still, because this week he used either his pointer finger or thumb to grab an individual string. I was focusing on singing D and A (the second highest and highest string) as we plucked them to start developing an aural connection. Now that he is grabbing onto a string, I want to focus on having him pull it in a sideways direction so it gets a good sound. He also held on to the CelloPhant™ (the cello bow grip) in his left hand and we used a pushing motion to play each string.

I'm really enjoying working with Alex and I'm so excited for what's to come!

Hope all is well,

April

Of the many, many things that I miss about pre-pandemic life, April's emails top the list. It has been a true joy to be able to participate in Alex's cello lessons, but there was something about him having something all his own, without my interference, that I really appreciated—for him. When my other two were Alex's age, they were forever asserting their independence, letting me know that, though they loved me, they also viewed me as "uncool."

I liked that Alex had a space where he could develop an interest all his own. I could support it, sure—the way I supported Josh and Sam by going to their track meets and soccer games, respectively—but it could remain his, without any of my mommy-interference. Of course, I could and did bear witness to all of Alex's lessons by watching his lesson videos, often with Alex, but I think he appreciated his sense of independence and I'm looking forward to the day when he can be back working one-on-one with April again and I can witness it all through her insightful emails accompanied by precious, priceless videos.

Alex:

Today I plucked the cello strings all by myself. I can do anything when I am given a chance. Learning to play this cello makes me proud. I think my family is proud. I know my teachers and friends are proud. The other day one of my friends, whose his name is Alex, like mine, wanted to watch my lesson and Miss Beard let him. It makes me feel exceptional. I know my parents tell me I am but now I feel I am.

16   April

It was somewhere around Alex's tenth birthday that Nancy had the idea of watching the videos of our lessons with Alex himself, so that Alex could see himself reflected back to himself and witness his own progress. She sent me an email after Alex's tenth birthday celebration and wrote in response to two videos I'd sent her:

> Both vids were great!! This was a wonderful birthday gift!! Alex watched the vid and got extra happy for the Happy Birthday song. This has been a terrific day!!

Nancy is the queen of the exclamation marks, and her enthusiasm quickly became my enthusiasm. Reading her words, I was transported back to a time in my own life when I had the freedom to play and to practice, the freedom to see myself not only as a person, but as a performer.

After completing student teaching and my undergraduate degree, I was at a difficult crossroads. It seemed I had two choices: go out into the world, start teaching and start building a music program most likely somewhere in New York state—or, as I remember my viola professor, Dr. T, suggesting, "Just go play." This became somewhat of a mantra to me, like a soothingly simplified statement that I could say to convince myself to go do something totally daunting and nerve-wracking because, of course, that easy sounding idea to "just go play" actually meant that I could go get a master's degree in viola performance and dip my toe into the intense and competitive world of performing. I began to envision the time as two years that I could gift myself, to work on myself as a violist. Little did I know, I'd be working on myself as a teacher too—so much more so than I expected.

I decided to just go play, and I always approached the degree from an educator lens, knowing all along that the journey was all in the name of music education.

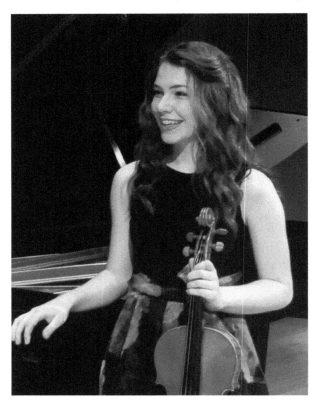

A post-performance smile after a recital.

I remember when I auditioned for the Metropolitan Youth Orchestra on Long Island during my freshman year of high school, and after playing my audition solo for the conductor, he asked me who my private teacher was. As I said her name, he smiled knowingly and said, "Yes, you play like her." From that experience I learned that students are mimics, so I wanted to become the best model on my instrument that I could be for my future students. If I could really hone in on my skills through struggle and process and work, I could simultaneously learn to better understand how to teach the skills I achieved. At the University of Delaware, I was extremely fortunate to be able to study with one the most beautiful violists I'd ever heard, and she taught me more about what it means to be a violist and a musician in this world than I could've ever thought possible. I was also lucky to be able to teach throughout most of the degree through a few different community string programs. This gave me a chance to apply the teaching skills I'd learned in real-world scenarios.

Looking back now, I see those two years as pivotal to my development the same way I see Alex's years of music education as pivotal to his. So much learning about yourself occurs when practicing an instrument. I think Alex has been able to learn a lot about himself through studying the cello, and—perhaps just as beautifully—so have his family, friends, teachers, and anyone he meets.

Reading Nancy's email about Alex's birthday festivities (watching him play Happy Birthday to himself), I started to think about how every musician has both their private experience and their public experience. We all have our own inner process of exploration and exposure. We go inward first, then we go outward, and share with others. Something beautiful and unique about Alex's experience of learning has been that he has been sharing the process with others throughout. During his lessons, he's had me, Kristen, Nancy, or Tracy assist him in ways that enable his learning and, yet, in watching himself, he was being granted his own experience of himself. Alex could see his musical gifts and talents, as well as his progress, and be buoyed by his own brilliance. He loves seeing himself and it's no wonder. The rest of us have loved seeing him, too.

17   Nancy

Over the course of weeks, then months, now years, April and I developed more than just a working relationship. I regularly wrote to thank her for her work with Alex. She regularly wrote to thank me for my support and to express her gratitude for how much my son has enriched her life.

Alex! Alex who blesses all who meet him. Alex, with his expansive smile and expressive eyes. Joyful, beautiful Alex, who is beloved by so many and, at the same time, about whom I often receive messages of struggle and sadness—or to-do lists.

My messages from April have been entirely different. One of the notes she sent contained one small but significant sentence:

> I will plan on videoing our whole lessons on his iPad because you never know what awesome thing we might capture!

I knew when I read April's words that these videos of Alex would become important in our lives. I had no idea how much magic they would generate.

Sharing these videos with Alex's GaGa was especially priceless. GaGa was always thrilled to see her grandson making progress, and asked me to send her a copy of each week's video. If I forgot to forward it, I would hear about it. Throughout her uterine cancer diagnosis, chemotherapy and even hospice, these videos gave her joy, and a sense of peace that cannot be put into words. Now, in addition to my heart soaring at Alex's continued expansion as a musician, there's a slight heartache at the knowledge that I cannot email visual evidence of Alex's progress to her. I know she knows, wherever she is, that Alex is happy and thriving and I sometimes sit with Alex in the garden and say a prayer in her honor while he looks at the sky, the same way he used to look up at her shining, smiling face.

I also share Alex's lesson videos with my mom, Alex's Grandma JoAnne, and she lights up at them. Grandma JoAnne had to be hospitalized briefly, and, when Josh, my first son, and I visited her in

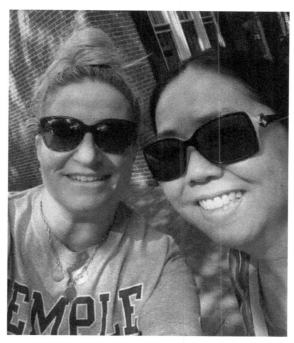

Noriko and Nancy at Michael's (Alex's dad's) art show on the Brandywine River. Noriko has been a brilliant support in the final editing of this book.

the hospital, Josh showed her Alex's cello lesson from that week. Her tears of joy made us all teary. Friends still comment on videos of the cello lesson I have shared with them. When I shared with my friend, Noriko, that I was writing this book, she remarked on the beautiful symbiosis the lessons show between Alex's learning, and April's teaching. She is absolutely right. I love each video. I can see Alex's progress, I can see April's gifted teaching, and I am filled with hope. These days, I get to see the lessons live and to participate in them because I am Alex's lesson assistant, and still I am in awe.

During the lessons, April emphasizes what Alex *can* do, not what he cannot do yet. She amplifies the positive. Every child needs this type of instruction. It is inspiring. On a day when Alex has had a nocturnal seizure the night before, or he is sad, or he cannot convey in words a need to use the facilities, or is having an off day, April still sees the things he does well and praises him for that. She is a powerful educator who finds and supports his gifts, and the more she acknowledges him for being where he is, the more he has been able to move forward into previously unimagined possibilities.

I think, sometimes, life is preparing us in the present moment for future experiences we could never possibly anticipate. It was only as April and I began writing this book that it occurred to me that, if I had not had my own experiences with stringed instruments, I would not have been able to support my son in his musical evolution.

With the power of hindsight, I can see that not only is Alex the son my soul needed—like my other two beautiful sons Josh and Sam who came before him—but I am uniquely equipped to be Alex's mother. Our relationship feels like a beautiful symphony, each instrument playing its part, everything in perfect harmony.

My youngest son has given so much to my life, in the overt ways that he, as a person, contributes to my life by being adorable, bright, funny, kind, gentle and all the qualities that draw me and others to him. And, at the same time, Alex has made me a better person—a better mother, teacher, daughter, wife, sister, and friend. Raising Alex has taught me innumerable lessons, and, although I could never capture all of them, I thought I'd share ten that make my heart sing:

- Inclusion does not only happen in the classroom. It happens on the playground, in the hallway, at the lunch table, in the swimming pool, at birthday parties, during school board meetings, during extracurricular activities, and in the community.

- Patience is essential. Having patience with ourselves and others creates openings for connection and community. In this fast-paced world, it's in the slow, still moments that we discover the beauty in each other.

- Just because a person cannot speak does not mean they cannot understand or communicate.

- What others think is none of my business. Letting go of caring about the opinions of others is the ultimate lesson in personal empowerment.

- Our light gives light to others.

- Anything is possible.

- We owe it to ourselves and each other to express what is in our heart, and to always be authentic. This may be simple, but it requires courage to lead with our true selves.

- It's important to stay positive, even in the midst of adversity.

- Extraordinary teachers are everywhere.
- Love is the answer to everything.

Alex:

Why is everyone home? Now I only see my cello teacher on Zoom. I miss being with her in person, and I miss my other teachers. I miss my friends. I hate the mask my parents put on me when we go outside our home. Why is this happening? I miss being on the bus and spending time at school. I am tired of doing all of my lessons on Zoom. Zoom exhaustion is real. I feel like it may make my seizures worse because of all the screen time. I hope things get back to how they were, and I can do my cello lessons in person. I guess it is good I can still do them. Mom seems to like learning the things Miss Beard continues to introduce to me. Mom really likes learning the difference between up bow and down bow. I think she had trouble with that when she studied the cello.

18 April

Halfway through Alex's first year, I had a revelation. As Alex and I were navigating through the course of our planned lesson, I noticed that he was anticipating the down to up bow changes with movement with his eyes and head. I began to ask him "Which direction do we move next?" and he showed me—either using his eyes or his head. We moved the bow in the direction he indicated.

Alex began to show me how to use his communication to inform our actions and direction. We found a distinct language, as discernable to me as sheet music. Since that day, even before Alex received his Tobii, he and I have had the capacity to communicate in an unambiguous, direct and connected way. That was when we really hit our stride.

I expressed this to Nancy and emailed her along with that week's video and she responded:

> Hi April,
>
> This lesson was one of the most beautiful things I have ever seen. You can see the passion for learning Alex has, and the gifted teaching you bring, along with Kristen's amazing support. I just love, and look forward each week to your email, and video. Thank you for never giving up, and for always believing Alex CAN learn, and do things like any child.
>
> I saw the eye and head move in anticipation of your directions. I loved how you turned it to a question. Evidence of powerful teaching, and learning! He seems to love holding the bow, and making the gorgeous sounds on the cello. I love how he moves your hand to strum, and he does really seem more confident, and proud. At a few points when you said, good, or complimented him, I saw him smile. This is priceless. His smile does not easily come, and I cannot thank you enough for bringing it out like the sunshine. He truly loves learning with

you, since this is the end of the day, and he does not complain or cry, I know he LOVES his lessons with you!!

It is great that he is learning pizzicato with you. I bet he would love to hear you play some time too.

This is a definite turning-point lesson!! Thank you for your extraordinary teaching gift, and I hope you know how much our entire family appreciates what you do!!

Have a GREAT day!!

Best,

Nancy

When I began teaching Alex, I could never have conceived of how much the cello would come to mean to him, just as I never could have conceived of how much my own falling in love with string instruments would give shape and substance to my life. But music, like love, softens us. It makes us smile. It animates the dullness that exists within us and gives a new perspective. Also like love, music emanates from us and radiates outward.

The only Alex I have ever known is an Alex of smiles—a gentle, compassionate, heart-filled student who is eager to learn. I get windows into Alex's life. Not doors. Certain of his experiences will remain unfathomable to me. Alex has grand mal nocturnal seizures. He endures tough physical therapy sessions, and pain from the constant demands to his body that come with navigating the world as a person with low muscle tone.

I look at Alex and Nancy, and I see some of the strongest people I know. Nancy tells me that music has become a touchstone for their family. On difficult days, or after even more difficult nights, our lessons are one small form of embodiment Alex can experience. Though I believe his cello lessons to be a vehicle for working on things like his strength building, eye contact, movement initiation, focus, etcetera, it is also important that I allow his cello lessons to be a place where he can let go of life's stressors and simply be who he is, doing something he loves.

There are those moments as a teacher where I can wonder if I'm getting through to students, and I have to remind myself that string lessons might just be a weekly 20 to 30 minute blip on their radar of life. While music is like the sun to me, many things in my life revolving around it, to many of my students, learning an instrument may just be a small star in their infinitely speckled sky. So, I think it is important for me to remember to not be diminished by that fact, but instead it can make me inspired to make that little star as bright and meaningful to them as I can, so that perhaps one day it serves as a guide to someplace really special.

Alex is often happy with his cello, but after a long day of school and multiple types of therapies, if he is sad or frustrated during a cello lesson, I don't get discouraged or take it personally. The most important thing I can do in those instances is to continue to allow him the opportunity to let the cello be an area in his life where he is always succeeding, always moving forward, always basking in his accomplishments. And that belief is reinforced when I open my email inbox and there's a message like this one waiting for me from Nancy:

> Hi April.
>
> THANK YOU!!! These lessons are the BEST!!! It was beautiful!!! I LOVE how he smiled at you. He had had some seizures, and was not feeling great since his neurologist increased his seizure medicine. Therefore, it is even more incredible that he was able to learn with you, without crying or sleeping. True magic!!! The bowing is gorgeous!!! LOVE the songs too.
>
> I hope you have a great weekend!!! Stay warm!!!!
> Best,
> Nancy

Alex:

Surfaces is playing loud on my Alexa and Mom is getting me ready for school. She is spraying Sun Bum 30 sunscreen on my arms and legs before she lifts me onto the living room blue chair to eat my egg and cheese sandwich. The scent of Sun Bum with its coconut beach smell takes me to the beach. The Surfaces song, "Keep It Gold," transports me and wraps around my heart. I move my arms and kick my legs to the beat. Closing my eyes, I can hear and see the sea with its waves crashing against the shore. I groove on to "Keep It Gold." "The sun is shining on your soul." Love this song. What a spectacular, soulful song!

19 April

Like Nancy, I am humbled by Alex's learning as well as by his teaching. One concrete example of something Alex has taught me is to accept where I am and to keep moving forward. I learned that when we began working on independent plucking on his strings. On our seventeenth lesson together, Alex, on his own initiative, perfectly fit his hand in mine so our thumbs lined up and we were plucking in tandem, rather than just one of us guiding the other's hand like we'd been doing. It worked so well, so I thanked Alex for thinking of that strategy. As we continued plucking together, I saw his confidence rise. He became even more independent and assertive when it came to bowing. He began to become rhythmic with his bow changes from up to down and down to up. He was creatively purposeful when he wanted to move the bow. Through independence and interdependence, Alex got stronger with his playing abilities. And through Alex's example, I find myself realizing my own skillset as an educator.

Though I have a performance degree, I do not feel like much of a performer unless I'm in front of kids. If I am to perform solo in front of adults on a stage, I "suffer" (a bit of a strong word) from something called "post-performance amnesia," where after I walk off stage, I cannot remember nearly anything that just happened onstage. I can remember walking out and bowing to the audience as they applaud, placing my bow on the strings, cuing to my piano accompanist for the first note and then...nothing. After that, blackness. It is a pretty strange and frustrating feeling leaving your whole memory onstage like that, but if I try to look at it from an educator's lens, I feel strangely lucky to have this conundrum in that perhaps I am experiencing something that many of my students may feel when they are put on the spot or put in front of an audience to perform—whether it be an audience of peers or parents or even just performing for me in an assessment. Perhaps it's related to adrenaline or the extreme feeling of vulnerability, a hyperfocused fear of being judged. When I watch these performances later on (because most are recorded), my external self looks as completely calm and "cool as a pickle" as my mom used to say. To me, it looks like I'm nearly sleep walking...or sleep playing, I should say. I'm certain that maintaining that level of calmness is much more of a struggle on the inside, but luckily I don't let on too much externally, which once again, I think is true for many of my students.

If I'm performing in an orchestra, it's a much more comfortable performance situation for me, which is why I love to share with my students the importance of acting like a big team when in their own orchestra rehearsals and performances. In an orchestra, little human mistakes can be forgiven easily because your teammates have your back; or, in other words, your wrong note or two gets whisked away in the blended swell of it all. Sometimes, when performing with an orchestra, there are moments when you may need to "fake it till you make it" and by the time you get back on that moving musical train, nobody notices your little forgetful or lost-focus moment that you just had. The stress of being under a microscope is much less present for me in that scenario. I've been very lucky to be able to perform in some amazing places with orchestras, like at Carnegie Hall and Lincoln Center for the Performing Arts in New York City with my youth orchestra when I was in high school, and, though still surreal to me, I was able to perform in several cities in China like Shanghai, Beijing, Xi'an and Wuxi with the University of Delaware Symphony Orchestra. By the end of the tour in China, I felt that our orchestra knew the pieces so well that we could really enjoy it and be in the moment on those amazing stages as we played. Although Alex may not have experienced what it is to play on stage with others yet, that doesn't mean he doesn't get to feel part of a musical team. Aided by his circle of supporters, Alex has also gotten to practice playing with others.

The sensation of playing with a "team" reminds me of one of the first times I had Alex play along to a video of an orchestra playing. We were playing a simple harmony along with all those other amazing musicians, and I felt like I could see Alex starting to feel that same in-the-moment, enjoying-the-groove sensation I've always felt when playing with accompaniment. He leaned back a bit, tilted his ears towards the speakers, and began to sway. He moved with ease and contentment as we played along, and his eyes even shifted so that it seemed he was gazing out to an invisible audience. He seemed to embody that feeling of being one with the orchestra, with his coordinated up bows and down bows bringing it all full-circle. I knew then that Alex had become a true musician.

That moment occurred during Alex and my twenty-sixth lesson together, which happened at 11:10 on a Monday morning, instead of our typical 3:10 in the afternoon. It was state testing day, so our schedule was different and, having just been taking a nap at school, Alex woke up to see his cello right in front of him. As he opened his eyes from his nap, seeing me and his cello, in a complete departure from our typical schedule, his face lit up.

"Hey, Alex!" I exclaimed. "Glad to see you today."

His eyes said, "Hi, Miss Beard. Glad to see you, too."

For most of that day's lesson, he was in charge of the bow. He held it excellently. I had tried putting some fuzzy pipe cleaners around the frog (the part of the bow where the hand holds on) to try to encourage him to keep a little space between his fingers and to try a new tactile tool.

As Alex and I played along to Mozart's *Eine kleine Nachtmusik*, I was holding the bow very loosely, to guide it and initiate some movement at times, but, for the most part, Alex was in charge. He was activating his arm to hold the bow to the cello and initiated a kind of short, bouncy bow stroke. I gave him the vocabulary word for this type of stroke exclaiming, "Nice *spiccato*, Alex!" My own personal goal for Alex for the year had been getting him to hold and move the bow independently, and I realized with a wave of gratitude that he was getting very, very close to my goal for him for the year.

In my email recap to Nancy, along with my reflections on the lesson, I told her:

> I noticed a big difference in his posture when we play without the recording and with the recording. Without the recording, he is focused and listening to the skill we are developing. He leans in and connects to his hands and the instrument. With the recording, he seems to let his creative instincts take over as he is a part of the music. I think this is true for every musician. When we work on the small technique etudes and studies, it's all about the focus and development of something small. When we sit in an orchestra and play, we need those small skills, but I find I feel much more a part of something big. All that just to say Alex is certainly a true musician!

Although very true, I thought my observation was a casual one, and, while I suspected that Nancy might appreciate it, I never suspected that it would spark an idea that would prove to be one more blessing of innovation and co-creation that Alex brought into my life.

20 Nancy

April's email about Alex being a true musician sparked something inside of me. I read and reread her words. With the recording he seems to let his creative instincts take over as he is part if the music. I think this is true for every musician. When we work on the small technique etudes and studies, it's all about the focus and development of something small. When we sit in an orchestra and play, we need those small skills, but I find I feel much more a part of something big. All that just to say Alex is certainly a true musician!

The email arrived a few weeks before my first book was published in March of 2020, just before the world shut down. Alex's lessons with April were a pivotal part of *Up, Not Down Syndrome,* and April had contributed to the project not only by being a major cheerleader, and all that she did to work with Alex, but she also wrote an endorsement.

> "The truth and beauty of Nancy Schwartz's words tell an ongoing story of love, learning, and the power of acceptance. All can learn from this family's boundless hope and from their source of joy and strength: Alex" —April Beard, Music Educator and Violist

April's words on the back of the book, much like her emails about Alex, made my heart soar. In a moment of inspiration, I wrote back:

> Your last paragraph made me think I should write a book about our lessons with you, and what we learned. If you still have my emails, and yours from this year, (your email with my responses) can you resend them to me? I am going to think about organizing a book with our emails, and the work you have done with Alex, It is truly EXTRAORDINARY!!! I think the title of the cello book could be called something like Playing cello for beginners or Up Bow Down Bow...

At that time, because my primary career was mother and teacher and I hadn't yet embarked on this writing path, Michael and I liked keeping a centralized source of information for Alex, so we shared a single email address. I tend to hold onto things, but my husband, being the opposite, cleaned out our email inbox—and outbox—I had no more access to the emails and wouldn't have been able to recapture what at that point was a year's worth of memories.

April quickly replied:

> Compiling our correspondence over the year will be my little project next Monday since I'm done with lessons after this week (except for Alex, we will have one more lesson before the summer!). I'm excited to look back and see all his progress this year! Should I send his cello home for the summer with him next Monday? I'm thinking he can stick with that size for next school year, but we can always check in on that when school starts back up.

She not only sent our emails back to me. She painstakingly catalogued and organized them and, within a few hours of poring over our communications, I realized that there was no way I could write a book about Alex's experiences with the cello without his teacher, April Beard.

Alex:

Music is a language without words I can be part of. I can see and hear and groove, and I don't have trouble standing, talking, walking or being by myself. Music gives me confidence and love with tons of sparkle. Sparkle is what life is all about. Moments of joy, little moments like when Mom leans our butterfly bush next to my nose so I can smell the perfume, and watch the bees hum around the purple flowers. The way my brothers, Josh and Sam, on their off time, so tall and handsome, lift me into the pool to swim with me at the gym where they are lifeguards. The way Dad makes delicious food and helps me with everything. These moments are everything. Music is love. The way our dining room chandelier shines with rainbows carrying hope everywhere. Music makes my body tingle with happiness, and love.

21 April

A few days after Alex's eleventh birthday, we played Johann Strauss's *The Blue Danube* waltz together. Alex held on to the bow for so much of the lesson. I could feel the music take on life and energy through his performance.

He kept his ears and eyes engaged. I thought about how, in the span of a year, Alex had cultivated more and more of a sense of independent movement. He'd moved from information to application, and I could see his hand muscles ready to go and initiating even the small motions needed to get to that next step.

It's not always linear. There is one lesson I can think of when Alex arrived with a dirty diaper, crying because he'd been without a nurse, and without the help he needed for the better part of a day. When it became apparent that reaching out for the cello was not an option for him that day, I put the cello flat on his lap so he could strum the instrument in a swimming motion, bringing his pool skills into the music room. Then Alex did a wonderful job of tapping his hand on the cello to the beat of an orchestral recording I put on. When we switched to working with the bow, we celebrated his strong air-bowing techniques when I realized adding the cello was just too much for that day.

Nancy's ability to support me in supporting Alex has been instrumental to Alex and my work together. When Nancy mentioned writing a book about it, I was thrilled—for her.

I had known and been working with Alex through the end of Nancy's work on her first book about Alex, *Up, Not Down Syndrome*, and in that book, she included a beautiful chapter about Alex's cello lessons. I remember being pretty flabbergasted that I was in a book at all! So when she asked if I'd be interested in collaborating on another book solely focused on Alex's cello studies, I was excited, but wrestled with the thought that I was not qualified or certified enough to do this. Even now, I have really only been teaching full-time for four years, so I constantly think, *That's not enough to make me an experienced source. I have no degree or certificate in special education, no years of experience like many other teachers do...*

Writing about my thoughts and methods with Alex's cello lessons has been difficult because, even when the words effortlessly flow—and they flow because I love teaching children, playing string instruments, as well as teaching music to children—I still struggle with feeling qualified to say anything at all. All of this is just what worked for Alex and me in his lessons, and it really took off and blossomed because of Nancy's support. I think a lot of young teachers experience this "imposter syndrome." The "What do I have to say that people, students, or parents will find important?" It's a difficult thought to wrestle with.

When you have a relationship with a student's parent like I do with Nancy, it helps with this immensely. It helps to hear how music lessons have changed Alex's life, mobility, and confidence for the better. It brings me so much happiness to see videos of Alex's grandmother, JoAnne, or his other grandmother, Gaga, now passed, who was kind enough to buy me a delicate silver bracelet and a beautiful black scarf which she sent along with a little note:

> Dear April,
> Thank you for the wonderful care and kindness you give to my grandson, Alex. Wishing you a Merry Christmas and a happy and healthy New Year. Fondly, Sandy Schwartz.

My interactions with the Schwartz family have taught me that my teaching is important. Music is a beautiful vehicle for so many things for Alex, but maybe most importantly it's a vehicle for love: a teacher's love of music and helping children discover their musical powers; a parent's love for her son and his abilities; a boy's love for music and making his family proud. With Alex's lessons, this all happens in little moments, and maybe the success and importance of those moments will bloom later in other ways you never even thought imaginable. There are thousands of extremely knowledgeable, experienced, and dedicated music teachers out there—in fact, they are working all around me right now. I hope to learn from as many of them as I can.

Working on this book has been a reflective experience for me. What have I done well, and what can I do better, what are my goals for Alex after seeing what he's achieved so far, and what are my goals for myself as an educator? If I have any credentials to qualify me to pass on advice to others, it would be to parents of children with special needs, and to children who think they could never play an instrument: just sign up for that orchestra or band program when the flyer comes home from school. See what happens. I bet maybe a little magic can.

Nancy and my regular weekly email exchanges stopped on February 25, 2020. It was Alex's second year of learning the cello. In the coming weeks, the COVID-19 pandemic would arrive and shift our lessons to a virtual format. Like all things with teaching and learning an instrument, we adjusted—we spun in midair and landed on our feet.

Right before the pandemic hit, Nancy had been attending Alex's lessons, so that kicked off our transition from emailing my reflective observations from his videoed lessons to pointing them out in the moment. I think it is important for both Nancy and Alex to hear my live and specific feedback and praise, so in a way it became a more immediate mode of feedback and communication. Since Nancy was with Alex and doing the hand-over-hand guiding in our Zoom lessons, I continued giving my observations, feedback, and praise from the other side of the screen. Though it was hard for me to feel the micro-movements in Alex's arm or hand, or notice every detail of what he's doing as the computer screen blurs and the sound cuts out, I tried to make sure both Nancy and Alex saw the wonderful things he was doing. Nancy supported him with positive feedback and directions too, and it was effective.

Just recently (June 2021), we had our first in-person lesson since March 2020. It was fabulous to see Alex at work with his cello again, not through a screen! His increased strength really impressed me. I was able to see the row of small knuckles in his right hand bending and activating more, which is a skill I've been hoping to see Alex develop over the years. His arms were frequently extended on his own, and his fingers were able to grab and pull away from the strings on his own. The increased strength and confidence in his sitting posture was much more conducive to having the cello in the traditional set up.

I am learning Alex's music. It is often upbeat, occasionally sad, other times contemplative. Alex is creating his own song, note by note, lesson by lesson. He uses posture, movement, support, ingenuity, and tenacity to learn, much of it all through repetition.

I see Alex supporting his cello like it's a dear friend, and initiating movement to express himself and make music. I see and hear Alex balance all his strength and flexibility in a thoughtful and controlled way so that his tone emerges clear and beautiful. These were goals Nancy and I set from the very beginning of Alex's musical journey, and his progress through his goals, and now beyond, is inspiring. We will still always cheer at every thumb wiggle, every string tug, and of course, at every up bow and down bow. But a musician's work is never done, which is one of the beautiful parts about music. The process itself is the destination. We evolve, we plateau, and we adapt and adjust. I can't wait to see how much more Alex can grow. There is no limit to what's possible! With each up bow, down bow, and *pizzicato* in between, he inspires all of us to discover and express our inner song.

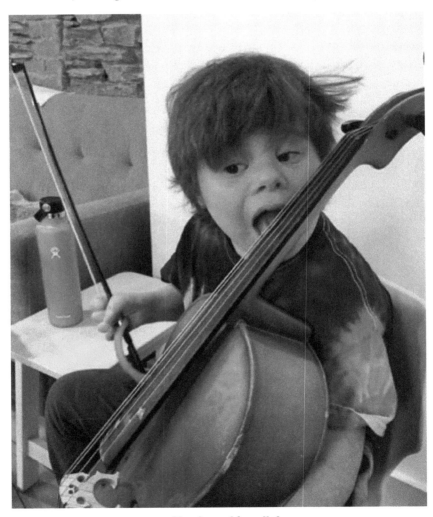

Alex loves his cello!

22   **Nancy**

As Alex's mother, I have occasionally found myself having to fight for others to see my son's potential. Throughout his lifetime, there have been those who have underestimated him. They've pointed out his limitations and challenges, and told me I was naïve to believe that his life could be limitless. But those people always have one thing in common: They don't know Alex.

Once people get to know my son, spend time with him, and see his tenacity in action, they tend to come to believe, as I do, that Alex's path will always be one of progress. Sometimes, this progress may be halting. There are moments of stagnation. But Alex adapts. He finds a way. He's been able to do that because of his own resilience and brilliance, and because of the support of those who refuse to underestimate him.

I thank G-d every day for April, as I walk by Alex's cello, which sits opposite his bed, facing outward on its stand, so that he can see it when he wakes and as he drifts off to sleep. As I prepare my son for a lesson, as I listen to Yo-Yo Ma, Matt Haimovitz, and others, or watch my youngest son groove out any time he catches even the faintest sound of music.

In the early days of April's work with Alex, and throughout their journey together, there were those who told April, "Don't bother trying to teach him the cello." To think if she, as a brand-new educator, had listened to the naysayers…Alex would not have had a chance to shine as the star he is. The brilliant little cellist with hopes, dreams and rhythms all his own. April's ability to see past obstacles, pain, trauma, and impossibility is an ability I wish all people could embody when they meet Alex and other individuals with Trisomy 21. It's a gift I wish all educators could integrate into their teaching philosophy, and one I myself hope to demonstrate not only as a parent, but as an ELL teacher.

After three years of working with April, Alex understands music more than most. He has an ear for talent, and the ability to put his passion into practice.

The benefits the cello have brought into his life are innumerable. He has grown physically in terms of muscle tone, posture, dexterity and strength; he has grown mentally from the influx and integration of new information; and he has grown emotionally. Once the cello entered his life, Alex's capacity for joy was increased. He laughs more now. And he dances a whole lot more. Sometimes, he'll use his Tobii to ask me to put music on. Other times, he'll simply gesture at Alexa with his eyes.

When the world shut down in March of 2020, Michael and I went into the same state of panic as everyone else in our circle of friends and family. We worried about the health of those we knew and loved, and those we'd never met. We watched in horror as the death tolls climbed, as people died from the coronavirus, and then from the brutal impacts of unchecked racism. But there was an enduring, unchanging bright spot during our pain, grief, worry, mourning for Michael's mother, and wanting the stress and the heartache to evaporate...

Alex's cello lessons kept us striving for hope in a trauma-filled world. The tranquility and solace that Alex's cello playing brings him, me, and the rest of the family cannot be captured in words. I can't wordsmith the beauty. You must see and hear it for yourself.

On March 21, 2021, April sent me a text message:

> Happy World Down Syndrome Day!!! I am sooooo blessed to have met Alex. He is the most magical student I could've ever asked for!! Thank you for all you do to make his musical dreams come true!

Her text embodies everything that I feel towards her, and I know Alex would agree. April is a blessing. She has not only given my son the gift of learning; she has given me the gift of witnessing his growth, a gift we felt essential to extend to you. In an effort to share Alex's music with the world, April, aided by Jason Zeenkov, has created a Vimeo channel to view Alex's lessons from the last two years of his cello study with her. Please visit www.upnotdownbook.com to learn more.

Even though Alex has challenges, as all of us have challenges, he's able to make music—beautiful music. Thanks to April's belief in him, and now his belief in himself.

Alex:

I watch the iPhone XS as Mom holds it for me. The video of me playing the cello fills me with pride. Me! I'm playing this gorgeous instrument and Miss April is next to me helping me play the strings with my bow. I love how we are working together to make this soulful sound. I like the position of my arms holding the cello. I can do anything.

Epilogue – Nancy

I like to say, "Challenge is an opportunity to be extraordinary." My favorite music activity is to play duets with Alex on our cellos. I never thought this would be possible. Alex enjoys the language of music now more than ever. Before cello lessons, I'm not sure if Alex felt the beat of music like a musician, but now he listens to music and bops along to the steady beat. I can't thank April enough for her bravery when deciding to teach Alex three years ago.

Gustavo Dudamel said in an interview on PBS, "Everyone deserves access to beauty." I agree one hundred percent with this concept. My heart is full of joy, as is Alex's, when we hear or play music together. This beauty is felt. It's tangible. Music is a magic miracle, uniting us in what's possible. Alex is thriving, and I believe one reason is because of his cello lessons with April. Alex responds anytime he hears music, whether it's at a University of Virginia football game, a Porch Fest while Jimi Kenrick performs, on a bus ride to school when his bus driver, Mr. White, plays pop music, or at home on his Alexa.

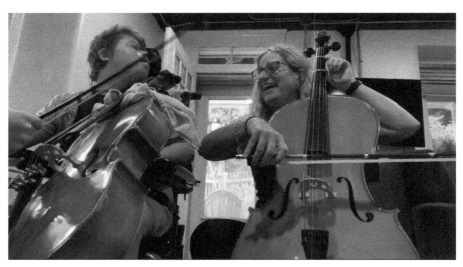

Nancy and Alex play a duet called Boogie Woogie.

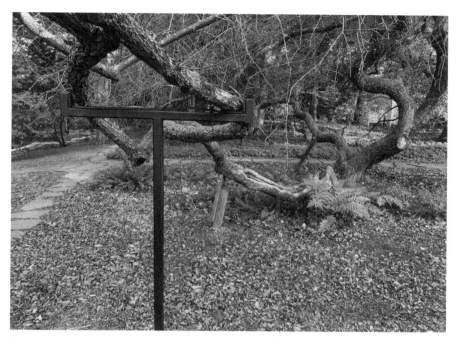

At Stoneleigh: A Natural Gardens, I saw this tree called a southern live oak (*Quercus virginiana*). Its metal support necessary for growth, reminded me of how Alex also needs support to grow musically.

The conductor from the Philadelphia Orchestra, Yannick Nézet-Séguin, said, "Music is mystical when words fail." Since Alex does not speak yet (I always say "yet" because you never know), music is a language he uses to communicate.

Shakespeare wrote, "If music be the food of love, play on." The cello lessons Alex has had these last four years are food for his soul and mine. April taught me that love and respect with high expectations is the only way to a true education.

Alex's Adaptations, Skills, and Goals

Here are some skills we worked on in Alex's lessons, along with a few adaptations we made to set Alex up to be successful. It took lots of trial and error, and sometimes things would work one day and not so much the next. Nancy and I continue to adjust his set up when needed. This is not at all a comprehensive list of skills and available adaptive tools/solutions out there, but just a few we found useful (or not) for Alex along the way.

Bow Hold: The cello bow hold should be as relaxed as possible. The cello essentially holds the weight of the bow while the hand guides it in the direction it needs to go. Natural arm weight is used to rest into the strings. The bow hold is where we've tried out several different adaptations:

- **The CelloPhant™:** a silicone bow accessory that goes on the frog. It looks like an elephant and guides students to make a rounded, relaxed hold. It also provides a more tactile experience for Alex, which can help him to maintain a more prolonged hold.

- **A pipe cleaner:** in his beginning lessons, I wrapped a fuzzy pipe cleaner around the frog to create a more tactile experience for Alex. We eventually switched to a half-size violin bow to lessen the weight of the bow and keep the length of the bow within his peripherals to support tracking of the full length of the bow.

- **A spiral hair tie:** a plastic, coil hair tie I found at the drugstore to use as a bow "seatbelt." I thought perhaps the coils would wrap over Alex's fingers and help him maintain the bow hold shape for longer, but I do not think Alex connected with this adaptation as much.

- **An EazyHold® grip:** this was a temporary addition to his frog. It is a silicone strap that is used for aiding in holding utensils, toys, toothbrushes, paintbrushes, markers—you name it! After removing the frog from the bow, you can loop one end on the stick above the frog, and then after re-attaching the frog, loop the other end on the screw so that it serves as a bow "seatbelt" (similar to the hair tie idea). Again, Alex has been doing quite well with independent bow holding, so I think for the time being it served more as a tactile grip, as he doesn't seem to need to put his fingers through the "seatbelt."

- **Cello Bow Force®:** a useful guide that straps around the C-bout of the cello. It attaches two suspended "guard rails" in which the bow travels a straight path between. This helps Alex see where to aim the bow to make contact with his strings, as well as encourages the correct right arm movement as he pulls and pushes the bow across the strings, parallel to the floor as aided by the bumpers of this training tool..

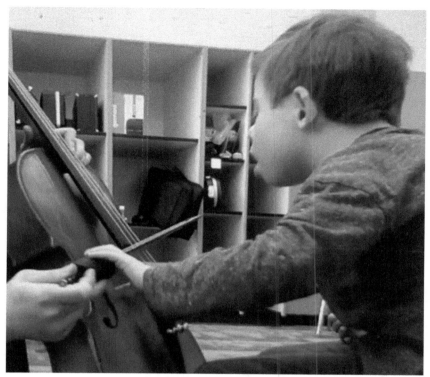

Alex using the CelloPhant™.

Bow Directions: In cello playing, the bow can be moved across the string in two general directions called "down" and "up." I think down and up bows are better described by the action that the arm has to do, "pull" and "push." With any of my students, I don't usually point out the down bow (or pull bow) and up bow (or push bow) directions until a few lessons after using the bow. I find that children naturally discover—without me saying much—that "what goes up must come down," and vice versa. For Alex, we practiced the movements of down and up bows for several lessons before I labeled the directions with their names. In classical music, bow directions play a fairly big part in technique and musical decision-making. Classical musicians will use the physics and dimensions of a bow in a very mathematic and scientific way to decide very specifically and with thoroughly thought-out rationale which notes in a piece of music should be up or down (In fact, I've witnessed quite a few hot debates on bowings among music colleagues). That's why it was so fascinating and shocking when I went to study Irish fiddling in Ireland during my undergraduate degree, and we discovered that Irish fiddlers really pay very little mind to deciding and labeling bowings. Instead, they'll just *move* in a way that feels natural. For Alex, I think we are somewhere in between these two realms of thought: we've labeled the directions with their names and practiced them using their names, but when working on some of our bowing music patterns, whichever direction Alex initiates first is great to me.

Note Identification—Identifying notes by seeing them on a music staff, or hearing them aurally prompted and then identifying the correct string on the cello. This is something we started in his second year of cello and we used an "alternative notation" (color coding). Notes on the staff are color coded, and we placed stickers on his fingerboard beneath each open string to coordinate:

- Open A is red

- Open D is blue

- Open G is green

- Open C is yellow

We also tried matching pieces of construction paper cut into square and rectangles. A square piece of paper would be a short note. A rectangle piece of paper (held horizontally) would be a long note. The pieces of paper can be arranged into a short pattern for him to practice watching and playing. Eventually, a goal I have for him would be to compose his own short pattern by selecting pieces of paper to create his own composition.

Patterns—we have found or developed several of these while working with Alex:

- **Rain pattern:** This pattern I got from composer Katie O'Hara LaBrie's piece for elementary strings called "Sky Suite." I was working on it with my fourth grade orchestra in 2020, and loved the second movement called "Rain." Each of the four movements was named after all the beautiful things that happen in the sky (I. Clouds, II. Rain, III. Thunder, IV. Sun). The simple bass line from "Rain" was a delightful addition to Alex's patterns and was a play on the sing-songy melody of "Rain, rain, go away" nursery rhyme. We played it along to the orchestral recording at a nice, brisk tempo. It goes: D A A A ǀ D A A A ǀ D A A A ǀ D A D

- **DAD song:** This is a beginner song for practicing identification of the D and A strings. It goes: D A D | A D A | D D A A | D A D

- **"Bach Pattern":** Alex loves J.S. Bach's Cello Suites, especially when Yo-Yo Ma or Sheku Kanneh-Mason play them, as Nancy and I would gush about in our emails. I turned it into an open string pattern inspired by the famous first suite Prelude. We practice sweeping the bow in a slur to connect the G, D, and A strings, then we "seesaw" the bow on A and D. It mimics the bow pattern at the beginning of the Prelude, while also teaching slurs, string crossings, bow control and distribution, and of course, coordination.

- **Open String Harmonies:** Alex plays the open string harmonies to many well-known songs like *Hot Cross Buns*, *Twinkle Twinkle Little Star*, and fiddle tunes like *Boil 'em Cabbage Down* and *Johnny Leary's Polka* (a fiddle tune some fabulous, young nine and ten year old fiddlers taught me in a study abroad in Kinvara, Ireland). The open string harmonies are a way to learn the bow rhythms and coordination of famous, well-known tunes. When I first started teaching, I was afraid these types of tunes would make my students roll their eyes in boredom or underestimate their maturity; and yet, I find that young students are incredibly motivated by these silly tunes! They've heard them a million times, they've sung them, danced to them, made memories to them, and they make sense musically too. Their form is memorable and predictable, and that gives young musicians like Alex confidence, because they are experiencing this highly-involved, asymmetrical, rhythm-driven, fine-motor coordination for the first time.

Pizzicato—to pluck the strings. When working with Alex on *pizzicato,* we work on finding finger action in the knuckles. After working on the motion of plucking with Alex, our goal is to see Alex initiate movements in his knuckles to tug at the string and produce a pitch. In several lessons, Alex did this after guiding his thumb to rest on the fingerboard.

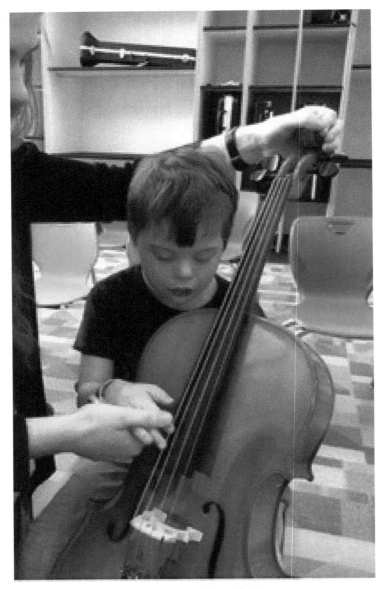

Alex practicing *pizzicato*.

Acknowledgements

Nancy:

Thank you to G-d (as part of my upbringing and honoring of the divine, I never write the name in full) for the blessing of my family, the ability to write, for music, for teachers like April, for friends, and for life. Thank you to April, my co-author, for her courage, support, and ability to educate.

Thank you to my husband, best friend, and co-pilot, Michael Scott Schwartz (*Shmuel*, his Hebrew name). The way he cares for our family, and for me, is everything. Michael inspires me with his creative spirit, art, intelligence, calmness, and sense of humor. What a blessing to have him as my partner. A unique thank you to each of my children: Joshua Owen Schwartz (*Baruch*, his Hebrew name), Samuel Zane Schwartz (*Moshe*, Hebrew name), and Alexander Gunnar Schwartz (*Gal*, his Hebrew name). They make my rainbow (*Koshti*, which also happens to be my Hebrew name) brighter, happier, and blessed.

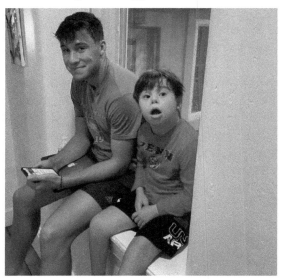

Sam and Alex at hanging out at home.

Josh is handsome, smart, funny, artistic, and caring. I am lucky to call him my son. He read this book early and made helpful comments and, every day, he makes me be a better version of myself.

Sam is gorgeous, disciplined, clever, witty, and kind. He inspires me to work harder and be strong. His work in school and on the soccer field is inspiring. It is a blessing to have Sam as my son.

Alex is beautiful, precious, smart, loving, and has a great sense of humor like Josh and Sam. They inspire me to try new things, and be a better person.

Thank you to my mom, JoAnne Liebenberg Levine for teaching me to love everyone, be kind, respect everyone, be optimistic, appreciate life, and to write thank you notes. Her appreciation of literature and music has inspired me to play music and write, and her love and encouragement are a daily source of strength.

Thank you to my dad, Martin Levine, for teaching me to be brave, strong, appreciate life, our differences and similarities, for giving me a Jewish/Hebrew education at such an early age at Forman Day School, for his love of great music and literature, and for his love and encouragement.

Thank you to my sisters, Wendy and Susie, for teaching me about love, and friendship. I hope Wendy is at peace on the other side. Thank you to Susie for her love, encouragement, and reading many drafts of this book.

Thank you to my friend, Noriko Lovasz, for editing the book, and to my friends Sharon Zeenkov, Elizabeth Castiglione, Beth Nordman Schoenlank, and friends too numerous to name. I am grateful for their love, and light.

Thank you to Michael's parents, Sandy and Lenny Schwartz, for their love of family, sense of humor, support, encouragement, and love. Thank you to Allen Liss for his love, support, and kindness. Thank you to Paige Figi, her daughter Charlotte, and her entire family. Charlotte helped to change our world in ways that are too numerous to convey. We lost her too early. I am thankful for her extraordinary precious life, and what she taught me.

Thank you to Barbara Bowman for her love and support. Thank you to Lisa Kohn for inspiring me.

Thank you to my readers. Thanks to the Gryphon Café in Wayne, for once again providing an inspiring place to write this book, along with community, and countless coconut lattes with a skosh of rose lavender, and super lemony water.

I am thankful to all of Alex's therapists and teachers, who have been with him throughout the years and make it possible for Alex to thrive. Thank you Megan Sabia, Kim Gambone, Kristen Culligan, Barbara Davis, and especially April Beard. I am grateful to Jason Zeenkov for his brilliant video editing of the companion videos, and for providing the incredible trailer for the book.

Thank you to the brilliant educational leaders that endorsed this book, graciously taking the time to read it: Barbara Bowman, Susie Garber, Russ Walsh, Brenda Dixon-Gottschild, Sharon M. Ravitch, Kass Minor, Betty Litsinger, and Jennifer Jie Jin.

I am grateful to my developmental editor, Daralyse Lyons, for her heart, incredible ability to lead, and her wisdom and insights. She worked tirelessly to fine-tune this book and make it what it is. I am grateful to my publisher, Victor R. Volkman at Modern History Press, for believing once again in the power of Alex's story.

April:

Thank you to Nancy, whose endless support, encouragement, wisdom, belief and love for her children and their growth has inspired me to become a better educator. I am so grateful for all of my hard-working and talented students, like Alex, who confirm that teaching is my calling, and they are my biggest inspiration as they beautify the world with music, sharing their gifts with others. Thank you, Alex, for bringing to life my teaching philosophy, and for showing your peers, teachers, and anyone else who sees you, that any child can be a musical superhero just like you!

Thank you to my mom, who has so much love for education and teaching children. She courageously pursued her education and teaching career later in life (after having my brother and me!), and getting to witness that led me to strive to be as dedicated, hard-working and passionate about education as she was and still is. She is the reason I was able to pursue my dreams of becoming an educator. Thank you to my dad, who is a natural teacher of all things about life. Because of him, I know how to be a strong, kind, and helpful person. Thank you to my big brother Danny who has taught me to be resilient, and that sometimes when we fall off that bike, it's best to just laugh it off and keep riding on. Thank you to my "Poppop," who also is the wisest teacher of all things that make the world wind-up and go, and whose never-ending work ethic is inspiring. Thank you to my partner, Mark, for always making me smile and laugh, and for being my biggest cheerleader. Lots of gratitude to Maria O'Connor, a music educator who is all about providing both inspiration and opportunity. Thank you for helping me find and pursue my dream career.

And thank you to my cat, Marty, who has taught me, by example, how to change course in mid-air.

Thank you to Noriko Lovasz, who brilliantly edited this book.

All my gratitude to Daralyse Lyons, this book's developmental editor, and Victor R. Volkman and Modern History Press, without whom this book would have remained an unrealized dream.

Most of all, thank you to those whose example has inspired me to follow my dream. I've had countless inspiring teachers in my educational years: public school educators, my private lesson teachers, some truly amazing music education professors throughout my college years, and my incredible viola professors at the Crane School of Music and the University of Delaware. The words, knowledge, and influence of these teachers have been infinitely powerful in my life. They planted seeds that bloomed repeatedly and in different colors, perhaps even many years later, and then brought new musical life to others. That is true teacher magic!

About the Authors

Nancy M. Schwartz has taught in Pennsylvania and New Jersey for thirty years. She holds certificates as an ELL Program Specialist, Reading Specialist, and Elementary and Early Education educator. Nancy's undergraduate degree came from Temple University, and she attended graduate school at Saint Joseph's University. Nancy spent several summers studying at the Teachers College, Columbia University, Reading and Writing Project. She enjoys ballet, reading, writing, art, fashion, animals, acting, music, and most of all, motherhood. This is her second book. You can find more photos and stories on her website www.upnotdownbook.com.

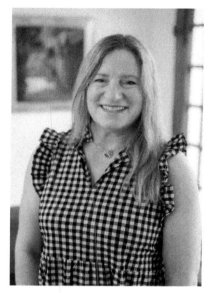

April E. Beard is a music educator and violist in eastern Pennsylvania. Originally from Long Island, New York, she completed her undergraduate degree in Music Education at the Crane School of Music at SUNY Potsdam. She received her Master's in Viola Performance from the University of Delaware. April looks forward to continuing to dedicate her work to sharing the beauty of music with children and leading them to find their own artistic success. When not teaching or playing her viola, she enjoys spending time with her fiancé, Mark, and cat named Marty, kayaking, and exploring new places.

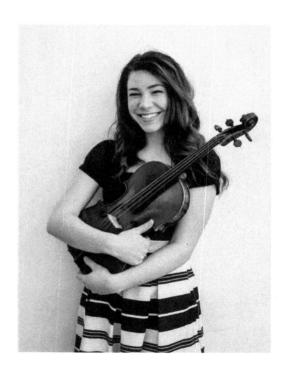

Bibliography

Albom, M. (2002) *Tuesdays with Morrie*. Portland, OR: Broadway Books.

Boushey, G, and Moser, J. (2014) *The Daily 5: Fostering Literacy Independence In The Elementary Grades*. York, Maine: Stenhouse Publishers.

Adamek, M., Darrow, A. (2005) *Music in Special Education*. Silver Spring, MD.: American Music Therapy Association.

Anderson, A. (2021) *Music, Sound and Vibration in Special Education: How to Enrich Your Specialist Setting*. London, Gr. Brit.: Routledge.

Calkins, L. (2000) *The Art of Teaching Reading*. London, Gr. Brit.: Pearson.

Calkins, L. (1994) *The Art of Teaching Writing*. Portsmouth, NH: Heinemann.

Calkins, L. (1998) *Raising Lifelong Learners: A Family's Guide*. DaCapo Lifelong Books.

Coelho, P. (1993) *The Alchemist*. San Francisco, CA: HarperOne

Copeland, M. (2017) *Ballerina Body: Dancing and Eating Your Way to a Lighter, Stronger, and More Graceful You*. New York: Grand Central Life & Style

Couros, G. (20215) *The Innovator's Mindset: Empower Learning, Unleash Talent, and Lead a Culture of Creativity*. New York: Dave Burgess Consulting, Inc.

Covey, S. R. (1989) *The 7 Habits of Highly Effective People: Powerful Lessons in Personal Change*. New York: Free Press.

Dixon-Gottschild, B. (2005) *The Black Dancing Body: A Geography from Coon to Cool*. London, Gr. Brit.: Palgrave Macmillan.

Garber, S. (2008) *Memorable Characters...Magnificent Stories: 10 Mini-Lessons on Crafting Lively Characters—the Key to Great*

Student Story Writing. Bethesda, MD: Scholastic Teaching Strategies.

Gelb, M.J. (1996) *Body Learning: An Introduction to the Alexander Technique.* London, Gr. Brit.: Holt McDougal.

Hampton, K. (2013) *Bloom.* New York: HarperCollins.

Hahn, Thich Nhat. (1988) *The Heart of Understanding: Commentaries on the Prajnaparamita Heart Sutra.* Berkeley, CA: Parallax Press.

Hay, L. (1984) *Heal Your Body.* Carlsbad, CA: Hay House.

Heard, G. (1995) *Writing Toward Home: Tales and Lessons to Find Your Way.* Portsmouth, NH: Heinemann.

Hugo, N. R. (2011) *Seeing Trees: Discover the Extraordinary Secrets of Everyday Trees.* Portland, OR: Timber Press.

Jellison, J.A. (2015*) Including Everyone: Creating Music Classrooms Where All Children Learn.* New York, NY: Oxford Press.

Irvine, J., et al. (2020) *The Karen Tuttle Legacy: A Resource and Guide for Viola Students, Teachers, and Performers.* New York, NY.: Carl Fischer Publishing.

Kieschnick, W. (2017) *Bold School: Old School Wisdom + New School Technologies= Blended Learning That Works.* Chicago, IL: Math Solutions.

Minor, C. (2018) *We Got This: Equity, Access, and the Quest to Be Who Our Students Need Us to Be.* Portsmouth, NH: Heinemann

Minor, K. (2023) *Teaching Fiercely: Spreading Joy and Justice in Our Schools.* San Francisco, CA: Jossey-Bass.

O'Donoghue, Jess. (2017) *The Observed Experience of Music Therapy on Parent-Child Interaction for Families with Children with Down Syndrome:* University of Limerick Library.

Ott, P. (2011) *Music For Special Kids.* England: Jessica Kingsley Publishers.

Polacco, P. (2010) *The Junkyard Wonders.* New York City: Philomel Books.

Ravitch, S. M. (2011) *Flux Leadership: Real-Time Inquiry for Humanizing Educational Change.* New York: Teachers College Press.

Schwartz, N. (2020) *Up Not Down Syndrome: Uplifting Lessons Learned From Raising A Son With Trisomy 21*. Ann Arbor, MI: Modern History Press.

Surette, K. (2019) *Creative Miracles: A Practioner's Guide to Adaptive Music Instruction*. Britain:Warrior Woman Publishing.

Suzuki, S. (1969) *Nurtured By Love: A New Approach to Education*. New York: Exposition Press.

Volvakova, H. (1994) *...I never saw another butterfly...*Washington, D.C.: Schocken;2nd edition.

Walsh, R. (2016) *A Parent's Guide to Public Education in the 21st Century: Navigating Education Reform to Get the Best Education for My Child*. New York: Garn Press.

Websites

www.noahsdad.com (Blog, Rick Smith)
www.charlottesweb.com (Stanley Brothers)
www.floweringhope.co (Jason Cranford)
www.TheRoc.us (Heather Barnes Jackson)

Twitter accounts that inspire Nancy M. Schwartz

@KOlusola
@sarahchang
@SharonRavitch
@YoYo_Ma
@GustavoDudamel
@PaigeFigi
@ChrisNikic
@PTXoffocial
@think_inclusive
@thekannehmasons
@HenryLouisGates
@NDSC
@IfWeKnewThenPOD
@DSiupdtae
@SpecialOlympics
@DSAInfo
@MindTendencies
@TheNapMinistry
@DrHoward_RECAST
@NDSS@pamallyn

@ernestmorrell
@MsKass1
@SallyDonnelly1
@ShekuKM
@charlottesweb
@realmofcaring
@InclusionEurope
@mencap_charity
@DalaiLama
@the stanleybros
@AimeeMullins
@ClintSmithIII
@Downsyndromecen
@DownDaily
@GDSFoundation
@NoahsDadDotCom
@DavidAgus
@TCRWP
@MisterMinor

Index

Up, Not Down Syndrome is a love letter and a map. Experience how it feels to think your life is over after having an unlovable baby. At first the loss seems impossible to overcome. Alex becomes the author's greatest teacher. Love is stronger than fear. Everyone has gifts. The book consists of three parts: the story, the lessons Alex taught the writer and Alex's perspective. *Up, Not Down Syndrome* is a promise to stay positive, no matter what: up, not down. Nancy's journey gets to the core of what it is to be human:

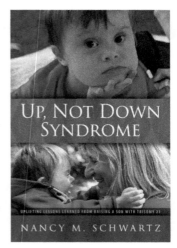

- Explore what it feels like to think life, as you know it, is over.
- Discover the fierce love, joy and peace a baby diagnosed with Trisomy 21 (Down syndrome) brings.
- Learn the lessons this child taught his mom.
- Understand the gift this baby brings to our world.
- Realize the depth of the love this family has for the child.

"A beautiful, honest account of not just accepting--but embracing--the unknown. Nancy shows us the blessing of an unexpected gift and the enormity of love." --Sara Byala, Ph.D.

"This is a wonderful book to remind you that the joy of love is possible in unexpected places when you open your heart to it." --Barbara Taylor Bowman, Irving B. Harris Professor of Child Development

"A moving and wise story of how a family navigates through hope, loss, learning and, most of all, love." --Rabbi David Wolpe, author of *David: The Divided Heart*

"The truth and beauty of Nancy Schwartz's words tell an ongoing story of love, learning and the power of acceptance. All can learn from this family's boundless hope and from their source of joy and strength: Alex." --April Beard, Music Educator and Cellist

Learn more at www.UpNotDownBook.com

From Modern History Press www.ModernHistoryPress.com

CPSIA information can be obtained
at www.ICGtesting.com
Printed in the USA
BVHW011129161222
654329BV00020B/1259